Eugene Salomon grew up in the suburbs of New York City, about thirty miles east of Manhattan, the son of an insurance salesman and a homemaker. He went to the usual schools (and to a couple of unusual ones, as well). After living in some of the more remote parts of the world during his teenage years, he returned to New York where he studied philosophy, religion, theater, and photography while supporting himself through an assortment of odd jobs. In 1977 he quit selling umbrellas on the street and began his higher education as a New York City taxi driver.

Confessions of a New York Taxi Driver

EUGENE SALOMON

The Friday Project
An imprint of HarperCollinsPublishers
77–85 Fulham Palace Road
Hammersmith, London W6 8JB
www.harpercollins.co.uk

First published in Great Britain by The Friday Project in 2013

1

Eugene Salomon asserts the moral right to
be identified as the author of this work

A catalogue record for this book
is available from the British Library

9780007500956

Typeset by GroupFMG

Printed and bound in Great Britain by
Clays Ltd, St Ives plc

FSC is a non-profit international organisation established to promote the responsible management of the world's forests. Products carrying the FSC label are independently certified to assure consumers that they come from forests that are managed to meet the social, economic and ecological needs of present or future generations.

Find out more about HarperCollins and the environment at
www.harpercollins.co.uk/green

There are certain rides in which the rapport between passenger and driver is so great that the only way to bring the conversation to a proper conclusion is a handshake. I dedicate this book to every passenger who ever shook my hand at the end of the ride. Except the drunks. That doesn't count.

And to Harry Gongola, Doctor of Chiropractic, former NYC taxi driver and my very first passenger.

Contents

Introduction

A conversation with the human race

A man jumped into my cab one night in April, 2008, at the corner of 5th Avenue and 57th Street. He was a forty-something businessman type, an *Inquisitario* (a passenger who asks a lot of questions) as it turned out, en route to Grand Central Station.

I could see he was a bit disoriented as he settled into the back seat, but this is not unusual in New York. Certain things must be confronted by a passenger as he enters a yellow cab in this city. Things like: how much will this ride cost? Do I have enough cash or will I have to use a credit card? Hey, what in hell is the source of that odor? And, since English is usually a cabbie's second language, does the driver actually understand a word I'm saying?

So it took him a few moments before it dawned on him. Leaning forward in his seat, he studied me carefully.

'Say,' he blurted out, 'you're an… *American*!'

'Yeah,' I said, 'but you know I charge extra for that.'

He ignored the joke.

'You're the first American driver I've had in... *three years*!'

'Better play the lottery tonight.'

'Really!'

I know how monkeys feel when people are staring at them in the zoo. There are indeed very few American taxi drivers in New York City. My passenger's eyes moved from the back of my head to my hack license.

'Eugene Salomon,' he said, not realizing in his excitement that I already knew my own name.

'That's me.'

'Tell me something, Mr Salomon... how long have you been driving a cab?'

'You don't have a heart condition or anything, do you?'

'No.'

'Well, then, I'll tell you... I have been driving a cab since... (drum roll, please)... *1977*.'

There was a short pause as this information was processed, and then the expected response: *'Oh my God!'* This is said in the same combination of horror and amazement people have when they see someone being hit by a car. I take it in my stride.

'Wow,' my passenger said, 'you must have some stories!'

'Buddy,' I say in a well-rehearsed reply, *'I have more stories than the Empire State Building...'*

The taxis

And I do.

If you make driving a cab in New York City your career you will get no pension, no paid vacations, no overtime and no health benefits. But you *will* get a collection of stories. It's inevitable. It comes with the job.

Why is this so? Let's take a minute to examine what taxi driving in this, the Monster City of the World, is all about. Especially if you're not a New Yorker (yet), a review of the basics is in order.

We are all familiar with the image of a street in New York that is filled to the brim with yellow taxicabs. It's a part of the landscape here. How many taxis are there? The answer is 13,237, a quantity that is determined by the city government. Why so many? (Or so *few,* if you've been standing in the rain for half an hour trying to get one?) Well, Manhattan, the borough where the great majority of these cabs can be found, is an island that is thirteen miles in length and two miles in width. One and a half million people live on this island and almost *none* of them own a car – there's no room for cars! So for many New Yorkers a taxi is a daily means of getting around town. Add to that the million tourists who are here every day and the more than a million commuters who are also here every day and you get an idea of why taxicabs are so important to life in the city.

In New York you can walk out into the street, wave your hand in the air (known as a 'hail'), and before you can whistle 'Big Yellow Taxi', a big yellow taxi will zip up to you and stop, making itself available for your grand entrance. Your carriage awaits you, sir! Or madam.

Consider how marvelous this is. What convenience! In most places you must call on the phone for a taxi and wait for that taxi to arrive, if it arrives at all. But the population of Manhattan is so dense that it makes the street-hail system workable. Hand goes up, taxi arrives. Amazing!

And the driver of that taxi is required by law to take you anywhere in the city you want to go. He cannot legally refuse you. Of course, it is an imperfect world and if you want to go to Brooklyn in the middle of the evening rush hour, you may be refused every once in a while. In fact, you *deserve* to be refused if you want to go to Brooklyn at that time! But, generally speaking, your driver will take you anywhere in the city you want to go. Again, this is an amazing convenience, if you think about it.

So we have here a system of thousands of taxis, all in competition with each other, cruising the streets and constantly looking for their next customer – anyone with his hand in the air. (Yes, I have stopped for people who were actually looking at their watches, pointing at buildings, or waving goodbye to their friends. And I have stopped not once, but twice, for a *statue* of a man hailing a cab on East 47th Street!)

The passengers

Anyway, who are all these people with their hands in the air? What kinds of people get into taxicabs in New York City? There are two broad categories: visitors and residents.

Who are the visitors? Well, maybe it's not *everyone,* but it seems like it is. New York has been called the Capital of the World, the City That Never Sleeps, Gotham, the Big Apple and other nicknames. As already mentioned, I call it the Monster City of the World. But whatever you want to call it, it is certainly a place where people from all over the planet converge. Sometimes I imagine that everyone in the world is standing in line in a single file. And then, one by one, they *all* get into my cab.

The variety is infinite. I am convinced that every conceivable type of person from every conceivable place is well represented in this city. From wide-eyed teenagers from Tennessee here on a school trip to middle-aged Barry Manilow groupies from England following the singer all around the country, or to an old couple from San Diego returning to the city after a forty-year absence – they all get into my cab. People from Turkey, people from Brazil; people from Estonia, people from Taiwan; I actually once had a passenger from Liechtenstein, a country in Europe that's so small it would fit into the *trunk* of my cab!

*

Most passengers, however (about eighty percent by my own estimate), are people who live in or close to the city. They can be broken down into seven main groups.

1. *The Workerbees* – these are the folks who either commute to and from the suburbs, live above 96th Street in Manhattan, or reside in the neighborhoods of the outer boroughs (Brooklyn, Queens, the Bronx and Staten Island). I define 'neighborhood' as a place where families live and kids can be seen playing with other kids without supervision. Due to the extremely high price of real estate, with the exception of the Lower East Side, there are basically no neighborhoods left in Manhattan south of 96th Street. The Workerbees I get in my cab are usually either en route to the boroughs or coming from or going to the train and bus stations of Manhattan.

2. *The American Aristocracy* – these are the people on the upper end of the food chain who were born into wealth and privilege. They live in specific places: 5th Avenue and Park Avenue between 60th and 96th Streets. Here we find 'high society' – prep schools, trust funds, debutante balls, charity events and the Metropolitan Museum of Art. And, yes, as a rule they are no better than average tippers.

3. *The Comfortables* – this group consists of those who are doing quite well, thank you, and can actually afford to live in Manhattan. They may have been called 'Yuppies' (Young Urban Professionals) at one time, but the truth is most of them aren't that young anymore. But urban and professional they certainly are. They can be found anywhere in Manhattan, but are most often in Midtown, the Upper West Side, Tribeca and Soho, with some hearty pioneers buying up brownstones in Brooklyn and Harlem.

4. *The Gonnabees* – it's been written that 'big dreams come to New York, small dreams stay home'. More than anywhere else in America, New York is the place where ambitious people come to make their mark. These are the Gonnabees. A Wannabee is someone with a small dream who stays home; a Gonnabee takes the leap and arrives in New York City come hell or high rentals. Most Gonnabees are in their twenties. The artistic ones can be found in the East Village, Alphabet City, the Lower East Side, and, currently, extending over the borders of Manhattan into the Williamsburg and Greenpoint sections of Brooklyn. The rest of the Gonnabees are pursuing careers in business and are sharing apartments in the Upper East Side or Midtown.

5. *The Unmoveables* – they can't afford to live in Manhattan, but they're too hooked to ever leave. These are the Gonnabees who never made it to the Comfortables. They range in age from thirty-five to ninety and could be anywhere in Manhattan, probably in a rent-stabilized apartment.

6. *The Flying Cosmopolitans* – wealthy, successful and smart, these are people from other countries or other parts of the United States who own apartments in New York but are here only occasionally. They could be living anywhere in Manhattan, but never in the boroughs. In fact, most of them have probably never even been to the boroughs except to pass through Queens on their way to the airport.

7. *The Flying Workerbees* – these people are working-class nomads from other places who are toiling in New York for extended periods of time and, in the case of Americans, may even commute back home on the weekends. They are either in Midtown or not far from Midtown. Both the Flying Workerbees

and the Flying Cosmopolitans aren't really residents and aren't exactly visitors either. They fall in the middle. But there are enough of them in taxicabs to be recognizable as distinct types of passengers.

The rides

So *these* are the kinds of people who get into taxis in New York City (along with an occasional dog). And what about the ride itself? What happens during a ride in a taxicab? There are three possibilities.

The first: nothing. The driver drives and the passenger looks out the window or watches the damned television which the city has mandated to be in the rear compartment of every yellow cab. The second: the driver is a fly on the wall. He finds himself the sudden observer of a scene in the passengers' lives. Middle-aged siblings are discussing their mother's medical condition and the driver is just along for the ride. Literally. Or two movie stars (Sean Penn and Dennis Hopper) hop in and talk to each other about – what else? – old movies.

And then there is the third possibility… a *conversation* takes place. And this is where it gets interesting.

Cab drivers and their passengers find themselves in a unique human situation. It's a business relationship but, like barbers and bartenders, it's a relationship that shares a close space for a limited length of time. Due to these factors the shell that divides strangers is easily shattered by the act of communication, and the potential for just about any kind of conversation exists.

Politics, sports, what's in the news today – these are common grounds for discussion, as well as the endless spectacle of whatever's passing by on the street. Of course, you never know where a conversation may lead you. Sometimes it may take you into something that might be called an 'adventure'. Like the summer day in 1984 when I picked up a man on 56th Street who was wearing white shorts and holding half a dozen tennis racquets in his arms. He turned out to be Martina Navratilova's coach and was headed out to Douglaston in Queens for a practice session. Thirty minutes later I am standing on a tennis court with one of Martina's racquets in my hand, trying to return the serve of a tennis pro. And Martina herself sits patiently watching as her coach has some fun with me.

Other times a conversation may flow so easily that the passenger and the driver find themselves talking to each other as if they were the closest of friends. I remember once bringing an elderly man, traveling alone, from LaGuardia Airport to Manhattan. There was a nice rapport between us, and this man told me about his life. He was one of the four Shorin brothers who had founded the Topps chewing gum company. He told me about the problems they'd had obtaining the raw materials used in making gum during World War II, and of the enduring love he had for his deceased brothers. 'It was one for all and all for one,' he said, as tears streamed down his face.

Others – on the assumption that the driver doesn't know who they are and will never see them again – will spill out their guts about things they probably wouldn't reveal to even their closest confidants. A man once bragged to me, for example, about how he cheated the city out of $80,000: he broke his leg at home but claimed he'd tripped at a municipal construction site and used his girlfriend as a false witness. Another time a man jumped into my cab in a true frenzy. Bouncing through emotions of anger and grief like a rubber ball, he wailed that he'd just been in a fight in a bar – and he thinks he may have killed another man.

Still others, trying to get a bargain by using their driver as a therapist, will ask for advice about anything from career changes, boyfriends and the stock market to how to buy a used car, how to make up a good excuse to his wife, or how to defrost a bagel. Amazingly enough, as years go by a taxi driver finds himself an expert in all these things and it turns out the passenger was wise to have sought his counsel.

So what it all comes down to is this: millions of people from every corner of the Earth - from Kathmandu to Katz's deli - are jammed together on a small island called Manhattan. They get into taxicabs and talk with their drivers. Communication occurs. And as years go by, a cabbie, looking back, will realize he has been having encounters, perhaps even *connections*, if not with every person on the planet, then certainly with every *type* of person on the planet.

He has been having, you might say, a conversation with the human race.

So jump in. Let's think of reading this book as being like taking a ride in my cab, except without the potholes. You want stories? I've got stories. You want opinions? I've got opinions. You want advice? Now why would you want *my* advice about… *that*? Well, since you asked, I happen to be something of a streetwise scholar on that subject, so my advice you will get.

But where do we start? Well, I think we should begin with the question every single person asks me immediately after they say, 'Wow, you must have some stories…'

1

The Wildest Ride

'What was the wildest ride you ever had?'

I have been asked this question so many times that you would think after all these years I would have a quick response to it. But I don't.

The problem is there have been so many. Was it the girl who rushed out of the cab seven times to puke? Or was it the guy who, without the slightest provocation, would just start screaming? Or the basket case who got out of the cab in the middle of the 59th Street Bridge? Or the one who got out in the middle of the Williamsburg Bridge?

Hmmmmmm…

Maybe it was the poor guy who was mugged while sitting in the back seat. Or the perfectly nice couple going home to Brooklyn who found themselves sitting between two cops who commandeered the taxi into the middle of a crime scene.

'Yeah,' I think, '*that* must have been the wildest' – but then I remember the ride with the Mafia hit men – and I just can't decide.

So what I do is this. When people ask me for my wildest ride, I ask them for a little help.

'What's your definition of "wild"?' I ask. This actually makes it more fun for me. It's my contention that I have some kind of a story for any category they can think of.

But I started to notice a pattern whenever I would ask this. First there is a pause. Then some giggling. And then, the BIG QUESTION: 'Has anyone had – *sex!* – in your cab?'

Always ready with a quip, my reply is: 'You mean *tonight*?'

'No, no,' they say with big smiles, 'ever.'

Soooo… *this* is what's on everybody's mind (surprise, surprise!). Well, who am I to deny the public what they want? What I'm going to do is rename this chapter. Let's call it…

Sex and the taxi

...and start all over again.

Okay, admit it. Sure you want stories about crime, hustlers, eccentric people and the gritty charm of New York City. But the first thing you want is sex. So let's confront this like adults, shall we? Once we get this sex chapter out of the way we can all breathe a lot easier and then move on to loftier pursuits.

So, do people have sex in taxis?

Yes. Not nearly so often as you'd think if you've ever seen the *Taxicab Confessions* program on TV, but, yes, it does happen. There are three stages.

1. *Cuddling* – two passengers get in and sit quite close to each other in the back seat. A head may rest upon the other's shoulder. There is some polite kissing. It's all within the bounds of acceptable public behavior.

2. *Foreplay* – there is suspicious movement going on in the rear. The kissing is passionate. There is no interest in any conversation with the driver. You look in the mirror and, where there were once two heads, there is now only one. They're doing

something with their hands, but you're not sure what. It's time to adjust the mirror and turn off the radio.

3. *Outright fucking* – if there are three and a half million people in Manhattan at any given time, then there must be something like two million beds. But apparently that is not enough. When a couple assumes the 'taxicab position' – the guy sits facing forward and the girl straddles him, facing the rear window – then you know they're adding 'taxicab' to their list of places where they've 'done it'.

One of the age-old questions is how should the driver react when he realizes that, only five feet behind him, and separated merely by a Plexiglas partition with an open window, the cucumber is entering the salad bowl? Should he consider this to be the epitome of rude behavior and throw the passengers out? Or should he take it as a compliment that they would feel so – what's the word? – *comfortable* in his space?

With me, I do find it offensive but my level of resentment seems to depend on the way the passengers go about it. While I've never thrown anyone out of my cab for this most out of place conduct, I do get annoyed if they're pretending I'm not even there. I have two ways of dealing with the irritation: 1) take extremely sharp left and right turns in an effort to knock the female off to the side; 2) charge them an extra ten dollars for the 'hotel room'.

So it's kind of oddly refreshing when a couple has such balls (sorry, couldn't help myself) that they make no attempt to hide the fact that they are intending to have sex right there in the back seat and they tell me so as the ride begins. It went down that way one night in the East Village…

Lust, cured

A guy and a girl came out of the Bowery Bar on East 4th Street late one night and jumped into my cab. The guy gave me their destination, 24th Street and 2nd Avenue, and moved halfway across the seat to make room for the girl. As she closed the door behind her she blurted out, 'You don't mind if we have sex in your cab, do you?' in the same way someone else might ask if it would be all right if she smoked a cigarette. Then she pushed the guy down flat on his back.

Before I could get the quip 'I charge extra for that' out of my mouth, she was on him like a Fido on a leg. It turned out it didn't matter if I minded or not, there was going to be a party on the back seat. Although I appreciated her outrageous effrontery, I wasn't too happy about having to suffer the discomfort I was already beginning to feel. But it was a short ride and I decided it would be better to endure it for five minutes than it would be to raise an objection. So we were on our way.

I drove half a block and hit a red light at the first intersection. As I came to a stop, I noticed something – parked next to the curb, immediately to my left, was a police car with two cops inside. There was a male cop behind the wheel and a female cop in the passenger seat to his right. Both of them were staring with great interest at the spectacle occurring on the back seat.

The female cop looked at me as I was looking at her. The expression on my face said, 'I am enduring the torture of serving in a professional capacity two animals who don't have the decency to care how their actions are affecting other people.'

I rolled down my window. She rolled down hers.

'Is this legal?' I asked, the tone of my voice implying that it would be great if she could find a way to bring a little justice to the situation.

She was right on it. She picked up her microphone (all police cars in New York have sound systems) and, with a big smile on her face, went to work.

'Hey, you back there in the taxi!' her voice boomed, *'What are you doing back there?'*

My passengers remained oblivious to the proclamation and continued humping on each other. People on the street, however, had begun to take notice.

'Hey, no sex in taxis!'

Now everyone within earshot was staring at them and beginning to enjoy the show.

'Hey, you, lady in the taxi – get off of that guy right now!'

The girl looked up. Suddenly realizing that she was making the day of about a dozen people on the street and, worse, was under direct orders from the police to cease copulation, she dismounted in horror.

'That's better! Now behave yourselves!'

There were still about ten seconds left before the light turned green. People near the intersection were laughing and one man actually began to applaud. It must have seemed like an hour to my passengers before that light finally turned green and they escaped from the scene of their public humiliation. And, you know, that little jaunt up to 24th and 2nd turned out to be as calm and sober as a ride to church on a Sunday morning with the minister and his missus.

Funny how passion can turn on and then suddenly disappear, isn't it? Go figure.

Awkward, defined

I was driving down Perry Street in Greenwich Village one evening when a pretty, blonde-haired twenty-something darted from the sidewalk and hailed me with what I noticed was an above-average determination. Most people just raise their hand and get in. This one was different – she had an agenda.

'Could you wait here for a minute?' she asked.

No problem. I pulled the cab into an open space near the curb and started the meter as my passenger-to-be returned to a townhouse and called out to someone. A second blonde emerged from the residence and was escorted to the cab by the first blonde. There was a brief conversation between the two of them and then, to my surprise, the front right door opened and the second blonde was ushered in beside me by her friend, who then walked back toward the townhouse.

'You're going to sit up here?' I asked the second blonde.

'I guess so,' she said in what might have been an Eastern European accent. She seemed a bit confused.

I knew something was up. This never happens.

After a few more moments Blonde Number One, who turned out to be an American, returned, but she was not alone. She had with her a good-looking guy – dark hair, about thirty years old. They jumped into the back seat and sat together the way lovers always do – no distance between them and their eyes locked into each other.

'We're going to Brooklyn,' the female voice from the back said. 'Seeley Street,' said the guy, 'take the Prospect to the 10th Avenue exit.'

I drove down Perry Street to 7th Avenue South and made a right.

'Do you want the Brooklyn Bridge or the Brooklyn–Battery Tunnel?' I asked.

'Whatever's faster,' the female voice said.

'The tunnel's faster but there's a four-dollar toll. Is that okay with you?'

No answer. The couple in the back seat had already reached the point of defining everything but themselves as the outside world and shutting it off. Which is to say, they were kissing, fondling, and doing *whatever* with significant energy. I started driving toward the tunnel.

I knew immediately that I had entered a twilight zone of human behavior. It's one thing to have passengers groping each other in the back seat. But to have passengers groping each other in the back seat while a pretty girl sits next to me in the front seat in what was going to be a long ride... now *that* is quite another thing. I tried to think of something to say to her to fend off what I sensed could become the mother of all awkward situations.

'Where are you from?' I asked.

'Estonia,' she said, in that accent.

'Estonia... Estonia... I know that's somewhere. Where is that?'

'Near it is to Finland.'

'Ohhhh... it was part of the Soviet Union?'

'Yes.'

*

Well, I felt I was getting somewhere. I could talk to her about what life was like in Estonia and what had changed since the breakup of the Soviet Union; we could chat about New York City; hey, we could even talk about Finland. Her friends in the back seat would settle down and the two of us up here could have a polite little conversation all the way to Brooklyn.

Yeah, right.

What happened next was the equivalent in the taxi world of being slapped in the face. Blonde Number One disengaged herself momentarily from her stud, reached forward, and slammed the partition window closed. This is a major faux pas as far as the driver is concerned as the partition is there for his protection, not for the privacy of the passengers – not that a closed partition window really offers any privacy, anyway. Under the circumstances, however, I thought it was perhaps not a bad idea and I decided to ignore the insult and attempt to continue the conversation with Estonia.

'Uh, so how long have you been in the United States?'

'A year and one half.'

'All the time in New York City?'

'For mostly, yes.'

'Do you like New York?'

'Yes, it is wonderful city, exciting city.'

We were approaching West Street, the major thoroughfare that leads to the Brooklyn–Battery Tunnel. The activity in the back seat had calmed down just a bit and could, with some liberal thinking, be accepted as just a couple of crazy kids showing affection for one another. They laughed and chattered and pecked at each other like two canaries in a cage. It was kind of cute in its way and it allowed the bland conversation in the front seat to continue. Block by block I was learning more about life in the post-Soviet Estonia. It was starting to sound like a place I might want to visit someday.

And then we entered the tunnel.

Apparently this is what they'd been waiting for – the Brooklyn–Battery *Tunnel of Love.* Blonde Number One immediately got herself on top of The Stud and went at him. Not in the more discreet taxicab position but flat out across the seat. Their thumping and bumping could be felt through the floorboard and her encouraging cries of *'Yeah baby that's it yeah baby oh yeah that's it baby!'* could be heard quite distinctly up front. There could be no ignoring it: the canaries were fucking and they were fucking hard.

I glanced meekly to my right. Estonia's eyes were staring down at the area around her feet in a complete non-confront of the situation. Her problem wasn't only her selfish friend in the back seat. Her problem was me. And my problem was her.

When two people are sitting together in the front seat of a car they are sharing a close, almost intimate space. That's why females usually do not sit up front with the driver when four passengers get into a taxi – the front seat is usually taken by a guy. It's just a bit uncomfortable for a woman to be sharing that close a space with a man she doesn't know. And what we had here was more than 'a bit uncomfortable'. It was right up there with the recurring dream some people have of walking down a crowded street only to discover that they aren't wearing any pants. It was at *that* level of uncomfortable.

Nevertheless I made a snap decision to tough it out. I would continue my conversation with Estonia. But I couldn't pretend that there weren't two people fucking just inches behind us. I felt it would lighten the situation if we acknowledged what was going on. Better to stare the tiger straight in the eye.

'Uh… so how do the three of you know each other?' I asked.

Estonia moved her eyes upward from the floor and looked out through the windshield toward the tunnel in front of us. She was coming out of her trance.

'In restaurant we work together,' she said.

'You're a cook?'

'No, no, am waitress.' She turned her head and motioned in the direction of the back seat. 'She is waitress also.'

'And *him*?'

'He is manager.'

'Have they been going with each other for a long time?'

'No, no, this is new.'

'So you had no idea they'd be doing… *this*?'

'No!'

So now I understood. Estonia was the unwitting accomplice of her sexually adventurous friend, as was I. With this shared reality I sensed that a small, yet perhaps meaningful bond had been created between us. We were both pawns in Blonde Number One's game and we had to support each other. I felt a stirring of affinity within me. Did she feel the same way? I glanced over at her ever so slightly. Was she smiling or was this the way her face normally looked?

I considered the situation. I'm a man. Generally speaking, I am attracted to women. There are two people in the seat back there making love as if to say that *everyone* should be making love. The attractive girl sitting next to me seems to like me, maybe. I'm single again. Hey, this could be a gift from the gods. Should I cross the line of professional conduct and make a move?

At the end of the tunnel there is a toll to be paid, so I slowed down as we approached the booth. Blonde Number One and The Stud used this opportunity to take a brief rest, their faces popping up with grins on them that I would have to say could only be described as 'shit-eating'. Then, as we picked up speed after the toll and were on the highway, they switched positions – The Stud now on top – and went back to work.

I knew I had only a short time to make a move if indeed a move was to be made because we would be at Seeley Street within five minutes. I tried to think of something to say or do that would give Estonia the idea that perhaps we should join her friends in this crazy, impromptu orgy. But I couldn't think of anything that wouldn't make me come off as a complete jackass, so I did what in certain circles I am well known for doing – nothing. Nevertheless I felt that if I could somehow keep the conversation going, who knows? It might lead to *something*. So I turned toward her with the intention of making words come out of my mouth.

It was then that I noticed that Estonia had found herself a way out of the situation. She did what ostriches have been doing for millions of years. She closed her eyes, tilted her head to one side, and seemed to be pretending that she was asleep.

Apparently the orgy would remain in the back seat. I put my eyes back on the road, picked up some speed, and said to hell with it, I'd rather keep my dignity and my professionalism. But, then again, if she would just give me a sign perhaps I could regain my dignity and professionalism, uh, tomorrow.

But there was no sign. The ride from hell went on like this – Estonia pretending to be asleep and myself looking for something, anything – for a few more minutes until we finally did arrive at Seeley Street. Actually I had a feeling of relief when we pulled up in front of their building as, thank God, the ordeal was over at last. Blonde Number One and The Stud pranced from the back seat without the slightest hint of embarrassment, all smiles. The Stud then handed me a $10 tip on top of the amount on the meter, a worthy gesture that didn't really make up for the stress I had been caused to endure, but it did make me feel a bit better about things. The best thing, however, was that I was rid of them and could get on with the complacency of my daily grind.

Or so I thought.

Like the trick ending of a horror movie where you think the psycho is dead but then somehow he's coming at you again with a butcher knife, there was more.

After a brief conversation with Blonde Number One, Estonia decided to continue on with the ride. What she'd thought was going to be a night of hanging out with her friends had become a sex party for them but not for her. So what was the point of staying? She'd rather just go home. And home, it turned out, was several more minutes into Brooklyn.

I thought she would move from the front to the back and make the whole spatial arrangement more comfortable for the two of us. But no – she stayed up front with me! Now it would be just the two of us alone in the front seat. What had been perhaps the most awkward situation theoretically possible between a man and a woman who didn't know each other had actually taken a turn for the worse. *This* was even *more* awkward.

I pulled out and headed for Ocean Parkway. It would be an eight-minute ride on that road until we reached Avenue P, where she lived. Once again, the tension of the situation gripped me. What was she thinking? Was her staying up front with me a clue that I was supposed to act on? What should I do? *What should I do?*

Well, I wish I could tell you that the ride ended in a mutually enjoyable fling that I could smile about when reminiscing about my sexual adventures. But the truth is a woman has to just about rip her clothes off and dance the hula before I get the message. Estonia and I continued to chit-chat all the way to Avenue P as if the debauchery we had just witnessed had not really happened. She paid me the additional fare and left with a slight smile on her face. At least it kind of looked like a smile.

But it wasn't all for nothing. In the course of the remainder of the ride I learned that Estonia, the country, is bordered by Latvia to the south, Russia to the east, and the Gulf of Finland to the north; that the capital city is called Tallinn; that most people are Lutherans; and that it's a great place to raise cattle.

Fascinating stuff. Really hope to visit that place someday.

Multi-tasking

Multi-tasking. It's a concept that's gained quite of bit of popularity recently. The guy with a cell phone in one hand, watching a computer screen, reading a report and eating his lunch – all at the same time – is an image of the modern age. Why should it be any different in a taxicab?

I was cruising in Hell's Kitchen at around 1 a.m. on a cool, December night when a short, thickset guy – pale, white skin, slick black hair, about twenty-five years old – hailed me at 45th and 9th. A skinny, black girl, somewhere between sixteen and twenty, I would say, followed him into the back seat. I could see by the way they sat some distance apart that there was no great affinity between them.

I started driving down 9th Avenue expecting to hear what our destination would be, but there was nothing.

'Where are you going?' I asked.

'Make your next left,' the guy said.

'Okay.'

I turned left onto 44th Street but hit some traffic halfway down the block. We came to a halt.

'How long you been drivin' tonight?' he asked.

'Since five o'clock.'

'Busy tonight?'

'Not bad for a Tuesday,' I said, 'but things get slow after midnight.' The guy was showing signs of being a conversationalist. I liked that.

After nearly a minute we approached the intersection at 8th Avenue, but there was still no decision as to what our destination would be.

'Go left?' I asked.

'Yeah, make the left and make another left a few blocks up the avenue,' he replied.

'On which street?'

'Whichever one you want.'

Now this was weird. I immediately began to wonder why a passenger wouldn't care where I was going. The first thing I thought of was that he didn't intend to pay me for the ride so he didn't care how high the meter ran. But this guy didn't appear to me to be a flight risk. He just wasn't that type.

I looked at him again in the mirror. I noticed that I could see him but not her. There are only two explanations for this phenomenon: 1) they are cuddling with her head resting on his lap, facing upward, or 2) they are *not* cuddling and her head is facing *downward*... and you know what *that* means. Based on my prior observation that there was no particular love between them, I knew it was number two – this guy was getting a blowjob!

Well, at least I understood why he didn't care where I drove. The girl, I now surmised, was a hooker. My taxi had been turned into a brothel and, although I might have had cause to be offended, the guy had shown manners by asking me how my night had been going, and that was enough for me not to take issue with his behavior. I drove up 8th Avenue and made a left on 53rd, not expecting to hear anything but some grunts and perhaps some squishy noises coming from the back seat. So it came as quite a surprise that he resumed our conversation when we stopped for a red light at 53rd and 9th.

'Hey, you wanna hear something wild?'

'Sure.'

He mentioned the name of a former US senator from the state of New York and asked if I was familiar with him.

'Sure.'

'Well, he's gonna get indicted. It'll happen in a few days.'

'Really?'

He then dropped the name of a well-known Mafia celebrity who was in jail at the time and said he was 'giving up' the former senator in a deal to get out of the joint.

'What did he do?' I asked, meaning the former senator.

'He's been working for us for years.'

I paused for a moment while I processed this information. Here's a guy getting a blowjob telling me he's in the Mob and has inside information that a former US senator from New York is connected to the Mafia. Uh… okaaay…

'No kidding,' I said, 'that *is* wild.'

'Yeah, you'll read about it in a few days.'

'Wow.'

I buzzed down 9th Avenue and made a right on 43rd. We hit a red light at 10th Avenue. There had been a lull of about thirty seconds in our conversation but now that we were sitting still Mr Horny Mob Guy felt it was time to start chatting again.

'You play the horses?' he asked.

'Once in a while.'

'Write this down – *Wilfredo Prieto*.' (Not the name he actually said.)

'Who's Wilfredo Prieto?'

'A jockey. 'Bout a week before Christmas he's gonna ride a horse at Belmont. Fifty to one, but he's gonna win.'

'No kidding?' I wrote the name down on my trip sheet.

'Yeah, he comes up from Puerto Rico every year and does this race for us, then we give the money to charity.'

'Hey, thanks, man,' I said, 'I'm gonna use this.'

'Merry Christmas.'

'Thanks!'

I drove up 10th Avenue and made a right on 52nd. By the time we reached the end of the block the ride and the blowjob were over. He paid me $10 for a $6.10 fare and then he and the girl left the cab and disappeared in separate directions into the night.

Well, I was set. This fare, obviously a gift from the Supreme Being, was going to turn into my Christmas bonus. I started figuring out how much money I would be able to scrape together and even borrow and with a firm decision not to chicken out on this I began my hunt for Wilfredo Prieto. For the next three weeks I searched relentlessly through the sports sections of the papers for any sign of a race with a jockey with his name in it, but Christmas came and went with no mention of the guy.

And it may come as no surprise to you that no former senator from the state of New York has ever been indicted for anything.

So as it turned out I didn't make a dime from the Mobbed-up, BJ conversationalist. It did, however, leave me with an important Life Lesson: never believe a damned word that is said to you by someone who is getting a blowjob.

For old times' sake

It is lust that keeps the species reproducing itself. But it is love, respect and honesty that keep people staying together as partners throughout a lifetime. So it's nice when you meet a couple who still enjoy each other's company after dozens of years. It rehabilitates the idea that we, too, if we're lucky (or skillful) enough may also have it so good. With that in mind, here's a different kind of story about sex in a taxicab.

I picked up a man and a woman at a hotel near LaGuardia Airport on a lovely summer evening in 1987. They were seniors, near seventy years of age I guessed, and were en route to the Sloan–Kettering Hospital in Manhattan. Through the course of conversation I learned that their names were John and Barbara, that they were now retired – he had been a banker and she had been a teacher – and that the reason for their trip to the city was to begin cancer therapy for John.

They hadn't been to New York in forty years, they said, not since they'd moved to California after World War II. But they had once lived and worked in the city and, in fact, they'd met each other here when they were both employed by the same company in an office near Herald Square. They wondered if it would be all right with me if, before we got to the hospital, we could take a brief tour around Manhattan for old times' sake to see some of the sights which had been a part of their lives so many years ago.

Would it be all right with me? Were they kidding? Anything that keeps the meter running is just fine with me, and the truth is I always enjoy serving as a tour guide. It gives some contrast to the usual A to B fares and provides me a chance to show off my knowledge of the city, as well. I got on the Brooklyn–Queens Expressway and headed toward the Midtown Tunnel. Fifteen minutes later we were on 34th Street in Manhattan, heading west toward Herald Square.

The Empire State Building is on the corner of 34th Street and 5th Avenue, so I pointed it out as we approached it, thinking that surely this would be a sight they would want to see. But John and Barbara had little interest in the majestic skyscraper. What they were really interested in seeing in Herald Square was the Chock Full O' Nuts coffee shop at the corner of 34th and 6th. It was there, they said, that they'd spent so many lunch hours gazing into each other's eyes over chicken salad sandwiches.

As we got to the intersection both John and Barbara were straining their necks trying to get a glimpse of the place. But the Chock Full O' Nuts coffee shop was gone. It had been replaced by a Gap clothing store.

It was obvious to me this was a major disappointment for them. That coffee shop had been an important landmark of their life together, and now it was just a memory. We continued driving west on 34th Street in a gloomy silence, but after about a minute John spoke up.

'I know what,' he said to both Barbara and me, 'let's go over to 31st and Broadway. If it's still around, there's another restaurant over there that's pretty special to us.'

Barbara smiled, as apparently she knew what John was talking about. I made a right on 8th Avenue and another right on 36th Street, and we were on our way. A cheerfulness returned to the cab.

'There's a Horn and Hardart over there on Broadway,' John said. 'That's where I proposed to this lovely, young lady.'

I kept my mouth shut. I didn't have the heart to tell them that the Horn and Hardarts were long gone. When we got to 31st Street we found a parking lot where the automat had once been.

The gloom returned. I drove down Broadway until we were approaching 25th Street, and then Barbara had an idea.

'What about Schrafft's?' she asked. 'There used to be one on Madison Avenue. We ate dinner there a million times.'

I told them I wasn't sure if any Schrafft's were still around, but it did seem to ring a bell in my mind that there had been one on Madison. It was worth a try, so I drove to 23rd Street, where Madison Avenue begins, and we headed uptown.

The traffic on the avenue was a mess, which actually was fortunate because it gave us a chance to examine every store and restaurant on each block as we crawled along. There was a sense of anxiety in the taxi as each new block failed to reveal a Schrafft's and, by the time we were in the forties, the anxiety was taking on the feeling of despair. When we finally reached 60th Street, and still no Schrafft's, the search was over.

'Could you just drive us over to the hospital, then?' John asked with a tone of resignation in his voice. I made a right on 68th Street and headed east toward Sloan-Kettering. I noticed in the mirror that Barbara was dabbing at her eyes with a tissue. We drove a couple of blocks. Then suddenly John's voice returned with a new vitality.

'What about the Plaza?' he asked. '*That's* still there, isn't it?'

'Sure,' I replied.

'Well, let's go!'

*

Instantly their spirits lifted. The Plaza Hotel was only a few blocks away. I made a couple of turns and in less than two minutes we were parked right in front of the beautiful, old landmark. Both John and Barbara seemed mesmerized by the sight of it, almost in a state of awe. I noticed that Barbara's eyes were tearing again, but this time she made no attempt to dry them. John appeared to be getting a bit misty, too.

'We spent our wedding night here,' Barbara said softly, the tears flowing freely down her cheeks.

We just sat there for a couple of minutes in front of the Plaza and then John had another idea. 'Do you think you could take us for a ride through Central Park?' he asked me.

'Well, I could,' I said, 'if it's still open. They close the park to cars at seven o'clock.' It was nearly seven already, so I drove as quickly as I could to the entrance at 6th Avenue, and we were in luck – it was still open.

'Tell you what,' John said as he handed me some money, 'here's ten bucks. That's your tip above whatever the meter says when we get to the hospital. But the deal is, while we're in the park here, keep your eyes off of that damned mirror!'

Barbara scolded him, but I had taken no offense.

'It's a deal,' I replied. Some of the great events of history have been created by just such conspiracies.

We headed north on Park Drive, the road that runs the two and a half mile length of Central Park. The ride, with its scenes filled with trees, flowers, and people in each other's arms, took about twelve minutes. I must admit that I cheated two or three times and looked in the mirror to see what could be going on between two septuagenarians.

What was going on was plenty! They were wrapped around each other like a couple of vines and I would rank them right up there near the top of my all-time list of back seat kissing fools.

As we were approaching the exit of the park at Central Park South they straightened themselves up into normal sitting positions.

'I'm sorry,' Barbara said a little awkwardly, 'for using your taxi for a purpose other than the one for which it was intended.'

'Hey, that's all right,' I replied, 'cabs are for kissing.'

It was one of those brilliant utterances which come tumbling out of your mouth every once in a while, almost of their own volition, which are just the right thing to say for the moment. Any lingering feeling of embarrassment dissipated into the evening air and, as we came out of the park, there was a noticeable serenity in the taxi. I made a left on Central Park South and headed for the East Side. It took about five more minutes to get them to the hospital and, as we said goodbye, I sensed a kind of bonding with Barbara and John that I think was mutual.

I felt that I would see them again one day.

2

Big City Crime

Well, I hope you're happy. You wanted sleazy stories about sex in taxicabs and now you've gotten them – plus a nice, sentimental one I'll bet you weren't expecting. So now let's get down to business and move along to another much-requested type of story: crime.

'Have you ever been held up?' is a question I am often asked by passengers. After all, driving a taxi in New York City is a job that's more dangerous than being a cop and unfortunately we do often hear stories about taxi drivers who are victims of crimes. My answer to that question, which is, happily, 'No', seems to do little to cancel out the lingering suspicion in the minds of some that New York is an unsafe place. But this sense of unease is not really based on actuality. Statistically speaking, New York is one of the safest cities in the United States. What's bothering these people, I believe, is the perception of the *possibility* of crime. With so many iffy-looking people walking around, so many dark, deserted streets, and a media that heightens our fears with an insatiable appetite for crime, *crime, CRIME!*, we may lose sight of the fact that, generally speaking, people are getting along quite well with one another. But not always…

Swallowed

I was cruising along on West 75th Street on a pleasant evening in October, 1984 when I spotted a young man emerging from a brownstone, waving his hands frantically in the air, and calling out for me to stop.

'Please wait here a minute,' he pleaded as he came running up to the side of my cab, 'I've got to help my friend get down the stairs.' And then he ran back up the steps to the brownstone and opened the door there.

When I saw his friend my jaw dropped. He was also a young guy, medium in build, but he was completely covered in blood, his white t-shirt a red rag. As the two of them carefully navigated the steps and approached my cab, I could see that his face had been severely beaten, with his mouth, nose, and maybe even his eyes bleeding. He was indeed a horrifying sight.

'Please get us to Roosevelt Hospital as fast as you can,' the first one begged as the two of them slumped into the back seat. I tore out of there like the ambulance driver I had become and headed for the hospital, a sixteen-block journey. Of course, I wanted to know what had happened, and it was the explanation of the event, even more than the blood, which made a lasting impression on me.

What had happened was this: the guy had been walking on the sidewalk on the park side of Central Park West just as the sun was setting. There is a four-foot-high stone wall there that runs the length of Central Park, separating it from the sidewalk. As the soon-to-be-victim walked along, he passed another, somewhat larger, man who was leaning against a parked car. Suddenly this larger man grabbed him from behind and shoved him up against the stone wall. Behind the wall – actually inside the park – was another man who grasped the guy and pulled him up over the wall, into the park. The first thug then scaled the wall himself and proceeded, with his partner, to beat their prey to a pulp, as well as robbing him of his money and watch.

This incident became, in my mind, a metaphor for the condition New York City was in during those years. It was as if the young man in my cab had been swallowed by a monster – the city itself.

But by the time the nineties came around, the crime situation in New York started to show a noticeable improvement. Not only were the crime statistics down, the city actually began to *look* safer. Local politicians stood in line trying to take credit for the improvement, ignoring the fact that it was part of a national trend. But as someone who has been down in the trenches for a long, long time and as someone who might be considered to be sort of a professional observer, I formed my own opinion. Not to take anything away from police work that is sensible and on-target, nevertheless I attribute the drop in crime to three broader social factors.

1. *AIDS* – the devastation of the AIDS epidemic in New York City in the eighties and nineties should not be forgotten. I remember once having a passenger in my cab in 1989 who told me that he personally knew thirty-six people who had died of AIDS.

The two principal groups affected were gays and intravenous drug users ('junkies'). Well, guess what? The guy who broke the window of your car so he could steal the baby seat and whatever was in the glove compartment was a junkie. It may not be politically correct to say so, but if an epidemic is wiping out the junkies, the crime rate sure as hell is going to go down.

2. *The cell phone* – that's right, the cell phone. By the time the millennium passed, nearly everyone in New York City owned one. Today, if a person sees a crime being committed, he can immediately alert the police. I once had a passenger tell me that her nephew had been held up by a young thug who pulled a knife on him while he was walking down a street in Manhattan. As the mugger jogged off, the nephew followed him from a distance while calling the police on his cell. The cops showed up instantly and the thief, seeing them, tried to escape by running into a subway station where he made the mistake of attempting to sprint across the tracks to the other side. He managed to avoid the third rail but did not manage to avoid an oncoming train which struck and killed him. Not that the guy deserved to die, of course, but the truth is his demise did bring the crime rate down.

3. Now here's the big one, and it is surprising to me that I've never heard this mentioned as a reason for the drop in the crime rate nationally: *race relations are improving*. It seems to be human nature to become annoyed or outraged when things are going wrong, but to take no particular notice of it when things are going right. I believe the efforts of many, many well-intentioned people going back to the 1950s are bearing fruit – race relations are improving.

A kid growing up in the inner city today is not as likely to feel that, since he's not allowed to be a part of the mainstream of society, it's okay to commit crimes against it. He's more likely to feel that he has a part in the game, too. Due to a gradual leveling of the playing field in economic and educational opportunities, the boundary lines between the ghetto and the rest of the city are disappearing. It's no longer unusual for me to take a white guy to his apartment house in Harlem or to drop a black, urban professional off at his building in the Financial District.

But you're not going to see any politician get up and say, 'Well, the reason the crime rate is down isn't really because of anything *I* am doing – it's being caused by trends in the society that I have no control over.' To the contrary.

In the late nineties Mayor Giuliani, riding on a crest of popularity as a crime-stopper in his first administration, decided to take it a step further in his second and final four years in office. Seizing upon a dubious philosophy that if you can stop the little crimes you will also somehow be nipping the big crimes in the bud, he set an army of police officers out to seek and destroy sin at even its smallest incarnation.

Hounded

A woman of perhaps seventy years entered my cab one evening in September, 1998 whose destination was her apartment building on 96th Street between Central Park West and Columbus Avenue. In her arms she held a cute little Cocker Spaniel whose name, I learned, was Terrence. It took only a few words of admiration from me about her pet to set her off on a tirade. This woman was a firecracker ready to explode.

She told me she had started the day, as she always did, by taking her dog for an early-morning walk in Central Park. Not too far from where she enters the park, she said, there's a wide-open field where she lets Terrence off the leash for a few minutes to get some exercise before they head back to the apartment house. That day had been no different – she had let little Terrence off the leash.

But this is technically against the law and the violation was spotted by a cop in a patrol car who swooped down on her, she said, like a hawk zeroing in on a mouse. The cop informed her of the infraction and told her he would have to write her a summons for a hundred dollars.

Identification, please.

She didn't have any.

At this point the policeman could have taken her off to the

police station if he'd wanted to, but, she said bitterly, instead he opted to do her a 'favor' by hauling her and Terrence in the cruiser to her own building. After they rode up in the elevator to the 6th floor, she showed him the necessary papers, he wrote her out the ticket, and he departed, leaving behind one pissed-off septuagenarian.

One has to wonder what 'bigger crimes' are prevented by cracking down on old ladies who let their dogs off the leash. But one does not have to wonder why, after a few years of this, Mayor Giuliani's popularity plummeted like a stone and he began to be known as 'Mayor Crueliani' in my taxicab.

Upon reflection, I found that I had acquired a new metaphor. This incident symbolized for me what New York City had become – not quite a police state (thank you, the Constitution of the United States), but a too-heavily-policed state. The trauma of being victimized by a thug had been replaced to some degree by the trauma of being victimized by agents of the municipality itself.

But that is not to say that the city has become a place where crime is at such a minimum that you no longer need to have 'street smarts'. You do. And the most important street smart in a city of strangers is simply good manners.

The wrong guy

I had someone in my cab on a Saturday night in March, 1999 whom you know. Or at least know *of*. You have never seen his face, but you have wondered what he looked like. And you have spoken of him from time to time.

Let me explain. Has something like this ever happened to you? You are walking along on a crowded city sidewalk and you're in a pretty good mood, just minding your own business, when someone walking in the opposite direction bumps into you so hard that it knocks you off balance for a moment. You look at the person who did this and expect to hear some kind of an apology, but instead you hear this: 'Watch where you're going, *asshole*.'

Or this? You are waiting in line at the Quikcheck and someone a foot taller than you blatantly cuts right in front of you with his beer just as you were about to step up to the cashier. You think of saying something to the guy but he looks like a thug, so you just keep your mouth shut and stand there with your half-gallon of milk.

In both cases your urge to react in a forceful way is suppressed by the consideration of what the consequences might be if you did. You might be injured. Hell, you might be killed. You might be arrested and charged with assault. You might have a lawsuit on your hands. So you just stand there and take it. But you soothe your anger by thinking this thought: *'Someday that guy is gonna meet the wrong guy.'*

But the wrong guy is not you, so the moment of retribution has not arrived. Nevertheless, you know he's out there somewhere and it's just a matter of time before he evens the score with this subhuman who was just so rude to you.

It was the 'wrong guy' who got into my cab that night in March, 1999. I had taken a fare out to Jackson Heights in Queens at midnight and was heading back toward Manhattan on Northern Boulevard when I was hailed by a man who came suddenly running out to the street. I stopped the cab, he got in, and we drove off.

He was a stocky, Hispanic-looking man, maybe five foot six or seven, and he was in a state of extreme agitation. Without any prior conversation, these alarming words came out of his mouth: 'FUCKING BASTARD! DAMN FUCKING BASTARD!'

'What's the matter?' I asked (of course).

His answer startled me again. Not only because of what he said, but the way that he said it. He actually started to cry.

'Oh my God,' he sobbed in a lowered voice, 'I hope I didn't kill him.'

'What happened?' I asked.

'THAT STUPID FUCKING BASTARD!' he screamed. 'WHO THE FUCK DOES HE THINK HE'S TALKING TO? I WAS IN 'NAM, I DON'T HAVE TO PUT UP WITH THIS SHIT!'

'What *happened*?'

And then he began crying again.

'I think I killed him,' he sobbed as he covered his face in his hands. 'Oh God, I hope I didn't kill him.'

To say that this guy was upset would be more than an

understatement. He was riding on a wave of emotion that went up to anger and down to grief like a yo-yo, back and forth, and was literally inconsolable. It took the full ten minutes of the two-mile trip to Astoria for me to piece together what had happened.

He had been sitting in a bar, alone, just minding his own business, having a couple of drinks, and brooding to himself about his own troubles. Three rowdy young men entered the bar and sat nearby. One of these guys decided it would be a good time to have some 'fun' at my passenger's expense. He began making belittling comments to him while his buddies laughed. He wouldn't let up and it led to a brawl.

The fight was no shoving match. It became an outright slugfest which ended with the other guy collapsing on the floor from a chop to the neck which may have crushed his windpipe. He gasped desperately for breath before finally slumping over, unconscious, and possibly suffocating. My passenger ran out of the bar to the street and jumped into my cab which happened to be approaching on Northern Boulevard.

What the moron in the bar didn't know when he decided to forget his manners was that he had finally met 'the wrong guy'. His object of ridicule was an ex-marine who knew martial arts and was in no mood to take crap from some punk.

When we arrived at his place, I gave him this advice: talk to no one else about this incident other than a priest. Don't let your feelings of guilt put you in a jail cell. The guy muttered something that might have been a thank you, got out of my cab, and disappeared into the night.

I found it a bit odd in myself that, although my passenger had just committed a serious crime in the eyes of the law, I felt sympathy for him and was actually rooting for him *not* to get caught. This was partially because I had seen how remorseful he was and I did not deem him to be an evil person. But it was also because the person he may have killed represented to me an aspect of humanity that is begging for correction – the psycho who takes pleasure in intimidating strangers. This person, in my mind, is more of a danger to society than the guy with a short fuse who strikes him down.

Of course, New York, the city which prides itself on its variety, also has great variety in its types of criminals. There's the overt bully mentioned above; marauders who commit impulsive crimes like grabbing pocketbooks and running away; husbands who commit adultery; wives who put nail polish in their cheating husband's soup; and even the occasional sociopath who doesn't clean up after his dog (although this is rare, indeed).

But the one type of criminal we seem to be endlessly fascinated by, the one we can't get enough of, is, of course, the professional. Grouped together, they are the subjects of countless movies and TV shows.

You know who I mean…

They were hit men

These people don't go around telling you who they are. You have to figure it out for yourself. One Friday afternoon in February, 1985 I had two of them in my cab taking a trip to Newark Airport.

They didn't tell me who they were.

I figured it out for myself.

I'd been cruising lower Manhattan in the late afternoon when they hailed me from the street. One of them was tall and thin, the other shorter and a bit on the chubby side. They told me immediately that they had to go to Newark Airport in New Jersey; that they wanted me to take the Holland Tunnel; that they were getting a 5.30 p.m. flight to Chicago; and that they did this trip every week on Fridays. I didn't realize it at the time, but these bits of information were to become pieces of the puzzle needed to understand exactly who they were and what they did for a living.

I was glad to get a fare to Newark Airport – it was about a $25 run at the time – but I was concerned about the traffic. From where we were in lower Manhattan I would indeed have to take the Holland Tunnel and the rush hour congestion in the tube can be a nightmare, both leaving and returning to the city, and especially on a Friday. So I turned the radio on to the news station so I could learn as much as possible about road conditions in the area.

My passengers were engaged in continuous conversation, going back and forth from English to Italian. I found there was something about them which stuck my attention on them and aroused my curiosity. It wasn't just the Italian – it was a certain demeanor they had. When you do a job continuously over a long period of time, the types of particles you deal with fall into familiar categories. These two guys didn't quite fit. There was something about them.

I found myself wondering if maybe they were Mafia and I immediately scolded myself for even thinking that. I'm not the kind of person who goes around making bigoted assumptions. Still, I just couldn't get the thought out of my mind that they *seemed* like they could be Mob. It was not a thought I would normally have had.

Of the two of them, the one who really grabbed my attention as I glanced at them in the mirror was the taller, thinner one. He appeared to be in his late forties and had slick, black hair that was combed straight back. His face was noticeably pale and tight. This was a man who could have been cast as Dracula if he'd been an actor – he had a vampire kind of look. His companion was much younger, a bit heavy-set, with sleepy-looking eyes, brown hair and a protruding lower lip.

I engaged them with some small talk about the traffic. The younger one had some feeling in his voice, I noticed, but the older one had a voice and a manner in the way he spoke which I found disturbing. There was a hollowness and a solidity about him that wasn't quite like anyone I had encountered before. I couldn't seem to get free from an intuitive feeling that this guy was the real thing.

We approached the Holland Tunnel in traffic that really wasn't as bad as I'd expected and, as we entered the tube, the sound waves of the cab's radio went temporarily dead, not returning again until we were nearly at the end of the tunnel on the Jersey side. Then, as the radio kicked in, a story started to come on about a criminal trial which was taking place in Manhattan at the time and had been receiving quite a bit of publicity. It was called the 'pizza connection' trial because pizzerias were said to be laundering drug money. About twenty Mafiosi were being tried together as a group on various charges. As the broadcast began, the older one heard what it was about and jolted forward in his seat.

'Turn that up, please!' he blurted out in his heavily accented voice.

I turned the volume up. The latest details about the trial, which had been going on for several weeks, were given. For the twenty seconds or so that the story was being broadcast, my passengers both listened intently to every word. Then, when the piece was over, they sat back in their seats and began talking to each other with great animation in Italian.

As I turned the volume back down, there was something akin to a lump in my throat. I had suddenly realized exactly where it had been that I had picked them up – it was in Foley Square, the very place where all the courthouses were located. And they'd gotten in my cab at four o'clock, the time of day when a trial would be recessing. *And* they had told me that they make this trip to Chicago every Friday. They were going back home for the weekend until the trial picked up again the following Monday!

I knew at this moment as well as I could ever know that these guys sitting five feet behind me were card-carrying members of the Mob. Not Mob wannabees like the blowjob conversationalist whom we've already met – they were the real thing and were either on trial themselves or associated with others who were.

It took me a minute or two to digest this reality and still keep my eyes on the road. After a couple of minutes I began to wonder where in the Mafia echelon these two might fit. Were they big shots or thugs?

I ran that through my mind. I'd glance at them in my mirror and try to visualize them either as bosses or underlings. Did they give orders or take orders? I concluded that they must be low in the scheme of things simply because they were taking a cab to the airport instead of a private car. A big wheel would have some kind of a limo. But aside from that, how did they *seem*?

I looked at the younger guy. He wore an ordinary-looking leather jacket. He appeared to be a bit dull, actually. Definitely not a boss of any kind. I could envision him, however, as a muscle boy without conscience, perhaps hijacking a truck on I-95. He looked like he could play that part, but that was about it. He didn't have a perceptible sinister demeanor about him but nevertheless he was somebody who could inflict real brutality at the behest of others.

But it was the older guy, once again, who stopped me in my mental tracks. I tried to imagine where *he* was in the Mob. Possibly a middle-level boss of some kind, but without flamboyance or spark. I didn't find it difficult to picture him, however, knocking on a door which is opened by someone he's never met before, calmly pulling out a gun, firing it into the stranger's head, and then going home and enjoying a hot bowl of linguini.

The more I looked at him in the mirror, the more I became convinced that this was the guy. Yes, this *was* the guy! It was his manner, the way he carried himself, the way he looked when he talked to the other guy, the deadness in his voice, the shark-like quality in his eyes.

It is my understanding in life that people who decide to do evil things must first justify to themselves why it is okay to do what they do. What they're not aware of is that along with this justification comes an attitude. This guy had the attitude, just a nuance thing, of someone who had long ago justified to himself why it was okay to murder other people. It was *this* which was sticking my attention on him! I had never consciously observed it in another person before, but the longer he was in my space, the more certain I was becoming of it. I was driving a professional killer to the airport.

So how do you drive when you know that the fellow sitting just behind you puts bullets through people's brains for a living? Carefully! Two hands on the wheel, steady as she goes, and lots of space between the taxi and the other cars on the road! I figured the only danger I could be in from these guys would be if I had an accident while they were in my cab. We crash into another car, one of them ruptures a disc, and then a few months later, there's a knock on my door…

Fortunately we arrived at Newark Airport without a problem, a smooth ride that left them plenty of time to make their flight. As we approached the terminal it occurred to me that there might be one other little way of determining their status in the Mafia – the tip. A boss at any level would surely be a big tipper, right? But a triggerman monster would be someone who *knows* in his core that everyone is his enemy and no one really exists except himself, anyway. And this lack of empathy would show itself in the tip.

We came to the end of the ride. The fare was $26.90. The younger guy got out of the cab and the older one remained seated while he reached into a pocket to find his money. As he handed me some bills, he reached forward and put his hand on my shoulder (this cab had no partition). And then, while keeping his hand right there – *the hand of Death upon my shoulder!* – he said these words, slowly and strongly accented:

'I'm sorry, my friend, but I have not much money today.'

He had handed me a twenty, a five and two singles – \$27. A ten-cent tip!

It was an insult to my dignity as a working man. Hit man or no hit man, I felt I had to say something. I could feel I needed all my inner strength to say to him what I wanted to say, so I reached down deep to come up with the right words. And then I spoke those words with a smile on my face and without the slightest indication of insincerity in the tone of my voice:

'Hey, that's all right, sir, have a good flight!'

He closed the door and walked off toward the terminal. I pulled out from the curb and drove away in the opposite direction. Quickly!

Ah, the Mob. I've wondered from time to time what exactly the charm is about these guys. Why do we usually see them not so much as criminals but more as a form of entertainment? The answer, of course, is that we view them in the abstract. It's not really *us* that they threaten. They're either killing each other or some fool who was stupid enough to cross them.

One's attitude toward a criminal, however, can change rather abruptly when the victim is yourself. This was something I discovered first-hand on Christmas Eve in 1987…

The cab driver who does not speak English

As mentioned before, it's quite common in my case to have someone get in my cab and suddenly express amazement that I'm an American. Or, if they don't actually say 'American', they often say something like, 'Wow, it's really nice to have an English-speaking cab driver for a change.' Immediately following this comment I will be told a story about how my passenger was recently in a cab with some driver who spoke absolutely no English and had to use hand signals to make this driver understand where he wanted to go. I've heard this story so many times that it began to give me the impression that there must be a small army of cabbies out there who speak virtually no English.

And yet I had never met one.

It struck me as odd that with all these reports about cab drivers who don't speak English, I, who meet cab drivers all the time on the street, in garages, in front of hotels and at the airports, had never once found myself in a situation in which I could not communicate with a cabbie. Sure, there were lots of guys whose English was accented because their native language was Hindi,

Arabic, Russian or whatever, but never did I have to resort to sign language to make myself understood, nor did I ever really have a problem communicating with words. So what was going on here? Why do I keep hearing about cab drivers who don't speak English?

I had to become a crime victim myself to find out the answer.

On Christmas Eve, 1987, I was mugged. I had been at a party at a friend's apartment on 9th Avenue between 44th and 45th Streets with my wife and young daughter. The party went on late and it was after three o'clock in the morning when we were finally ready to leave. My daughter had long since fallen asleep so I decided to walk to 10th Avenue, where I'd parked my car, and then bring it around to 9th Avenue to pick up my family.

I made a mistake that I, as a veteran New Yorker and a cab driver, should never have made: I attempted to walk down a deserted street (45th), in a not-so-great part of town (Hell's Kitchen), late at night, carrying something that showed some value (two wrapped Christmas presents). When I was halfway to 10th Avenue, I was attacked by three thugs.

The whole thing took less than fifteen seconds: I heard running footsteps coming toward me from behind, I was shoved into a doorway, and I had a knife held against my throat by one man while the other two grabbed the Christmas presents and went through my pockets for my money (about a hundred dollars). Having gotten what they wanted, they then started to run down 45th Street, back toward 9th Avenue.

They say you follow your instincts in these situations, and my instinct was to let them get a bit of a lead and then run after them in the hope of finding a cop who could catch them and arrest them. I didn't want to get too close to them – they had a knife – but I wanted to keep them in sight. So I started running after them in pursuit.

When the muggers got to 9th Avenue they ran to the right and then were momentarily out of my range of vision. Then, as I got to the avenue myself, I saw them approaching 44th Street and run east on that street before disappearing once again from my view.

I stopped for a second and looked around, hoping to find a cop, but there were none around. I then realized that I was bleeding from the neck and that my shirt was covered with blood. Oddly, I wasn't terribly concerned about that at that moment. All I wanted to do was to catch these bastards. And they were getting away.

Suddenly I had a brilliant idea. I would hail a cab and then follow the thieves in the cab until we found a police car. I ran out onto 9th Avenue. *Yes!* – there was an available cab heading right toward me! My luck had turned. I threw both hands up excitedly to hail the cab and it pulled up next to me. I jumped in the back seat. This cab had no partition, more good luck because I'd be able to see the muggers more easily.

The driver was a young guy who looked like he might be Moroccan. He turned around to look at me so he could get my destination. I was obviously in a state of great agitation, but I calmed myself down enough so I could communicate.

'Listen,' I said, 'I was just mugged. The guys who mugged me are running down 44th Street. I want to follow them 'til we can find a cop!'

My driver did not react. He just looked at me.

'Go left on 44th! Please! Go! Drive! They're getting away!'

He continued to stare at me blankly. Then he started to speak. Out of his mouth came these words, and this is an exact quote:

'Obbie de bobbie de bah.'

I was completely desperate.

'Listen,' I begged the guy, 'I'm a cab driver myself and I just got mugged! Please! Go left on 44th Street! Go! Go! I'm a cab driver!'

'Obbie de bobbie de bah?' he asked.

I tried pantomime. I pretended I was holding a steering wheel in my hands and then pointed toward 44th Street.

'Obbie de bobbie de bah?'

Defeated, I got out of the cab in disgust, slammed the door, and walked back to my friend's apartment to tend to my wound. Although the cut in my neck had produced quite a bit of blood, it fortunately wasn't very serious and a visit to a hospital wasn't necessary.

The muggers were never caught.

I spent the following week ranting and raving to anyone who'd listen about cab drivers in New York who don't speak English. What's the matter with this city, I wailed, that they'll let anyone whose breath can fog a mirror push a hack here? Why should we have to pay good money to morons who think Madison Square Garden is some place where they grow tulips? Why, *why, oh WHY* does the Taxi and Limousine Commission allow these hordes of immigrants who can't speak a damned syllable of English to clog our streets with this morass of yellow clunkers?

And then I had a brilliant realization. I knew what it was! It wasn't that there were dozens or hundreds or thousands of cab drivers who don't speak English – it was this *one guy*! Everyone who's ever been in his cab is driven so crazy by this one guy that they start to generalize like mad and tell everyone they meet that there are no English-speaking cabbies anymore in New York City. But it's really just this *one guy*! Too bad I had to become a statistic myself to acquire such a profound insight.

It's just this *one guy*, I tell you!

3

Changes

I was driving a friendly, female Gonnabee to Williamsburg in Brooklyn one night in 2005 when she asked me that famous question: 'How long have you been driving a cab?'

'How old are you?' I replied.

'Twenty-five.'

'Well, then,' I said, 'I've been driving a cab since you were eighty-six in your last lifetime.' Which is my way of saying, 'Since before you were born, honey.'

Big smile and wide eyes.

'Wow,' she marveled, 'you must have seen *so* many changes!'

Well, the answer to that is kind of both yes and no. Certainly some things have changed. You don't dare light up a cigarette in a public place anymore, not even in a bar, or you will be immediately arrested by the cigarette police. The hookers have been driven off the streets (almost). And there aren't nearly as many New York 'characters' begging for our attention on the sidewalks as there used to be. (Like the 'Opera Man' who could often be found screeching out arias on the corner of 57th and Broadway.)

But for the most part I think things have stayed more the same than they've changed. The buildings are tall, the streets are crowded, and people are in a *big rush.* Donald Trump is rich and has a beautiful wife. And whoever was elected mayor has turned out to be an idiot.

The truth is I don't really know any more about what has changed or not changed in New York City than anyone else. Except for one thing – the taxi business. This is the one sector of life in which I proclaim myself to be the grand master, an all-knowing sage whose opinions must be given the utmost respect. So if you want to know what's changed in the taxi business, hey, listen up and take notes. There will be an exam the next time you're in my cab.

By around 1995 I became aware of an ominous trend which had seeped into the trade. People started to get into my cab, plop themselves comfortably in the back seat, and tell me they wanted to go to some destination in Brooklyn on the expectation that I would actually be willing to take them there.

This represented a significant change in the taxi industry. More specifically, it marked a change in the attitudes of drivers. Since time began, taxi drivers in New York City had been known for being crusty, hard-nosed men, often short on manners, fearless of authority, and willing to drive you to your destination only on the condition that they were in the mood to do so.

A ride to Brooklyn or one of the other outer boroughs at most times of the day is considered undesirable because it almost always means the driver will be coming back to Manhattan without a passenger – and that is dead time. So the driver sees such a fare not as money made, but as money *lost.* Thus he refuses the ride, even though he may be fined if the snubbed passenger makes an issue of it with the Taxi and Limousine Commission.

So prevalent were refusals to Brooklyn that the mantra of the New York City taxi driver had become – and this was a citywide joke – '*I don't go to Brooklyn.*' An old friend of mine who drove a cab in the '70s, Dennis Charnoff, used to claim that he *never* had taken a fare out of Manhattan. Not to Brooklyn, not to Queens, not to the Bronx, not even to the airports. Never.

In the spirit of the great talk show host Johnny Carson, who once joked that he planned to have the words 'Johnny will *not* be back after these messages' written on his tombstone, I myself have considered having the following epitaph written on my own grave:

Eugene Salomon
1949 – (a really, really long time from now)
TAXI DRIVER
'I DON'T GO TO BROOKLYN'

(Just don't bury me in Brooklyn. It would kill the whole joke.)

So what happened to the brassy driver with an attitude? What changed? The ethnicity of taxi drivers, that's what changed. By around 1995, by my own estimation, something like seventy-five percent of cabbies were from India, Pakistan and Bangladesh. They had taken the place of drivers from such countries as Greece, Israel, Russia, Taiwan and Romania. And, oh yes, America.

Why did this occur? Because the working conditions of the industry were allowed to fall so far below the standards of other available jobs in the United States by uncaring city officials that experienced drivers were leaving the business in droves.

In 1979 a change in the rules made all taxi drivers 'independent contractors'. (Even though the city retained the right to tell us what we may charge for our services. How 'independent' is that?) 'Independent contractor' means 'self-employed'. Thus, no benefits. No sick days, no overtime, no paid vacations, no health care, no pensions. Add onto that twelve hour shifts, a job that is dangerous, and no union to demand timely rate increases (yes, a workforce of forty thousand and no union) and you no longer have to wonder why you can't remember the last time you had an American at the wheel of your cab. Or a Russian, Israeli or Greek, for that matter.

The void was filled by the Indians and Pakistanis. When immigration regulations allowed these workers to enter the country and get green cards, the bosses of the taxi business discovered they had finally found the perfect cab driver – someone whose present working conditions are so much better than what they were in the old country (a Pakistani driver once told me he made better money driving a cab in New York than he would if he were a medical doctor in Pakistan) that he actually puts great value on his job as a taxi driver and will do whatever he has to do to make sure he doesn't lose it.

In short, taxi drivers have become compliant and timid. Gone is the guy named Lenny smoking a cigar who drops you off on Lexington instead of Park because 'Park is out of my way'. Gone is the maniac who speeds past police cars and runs red lights. It makes me nostalgic, it does, for the good old days…

Jackie oh my God

On a beautiful summer day in 1981, unfortunately with a passenger already in the back seat of my cab, I stopped at a red light on Central Park South, right next to the Plaza Hotel. Suddenly appearing from out of nowhere, as if from a dream, and walking right toward me was a sight that stunned me completely and utterly.

It was Jackie Kennedy.

I'm not sure if my jaw literally dropped, but if someone told me it was down on the floorboard I would not have been completely surprised.

'Oh my God,' I blurted out to my passenger, 'it's Jackie Kennedy!'

'Oh my God,' she replied with equal amazement, 'it *is* Jackie Kennedy!'

Yes, Jackie Kennedy, accompanied by another woman, was looking for a taxi and had sighted *my* taxi. Like most New Yorkers, I am relatively blasé about celebrities, but this was not just any celebrity. This was the *ultimate* celebrity. This was *Jackie Kennedy.* To say I was completely mesmerized would not have been an understatement.

Now you have to remember who Jackie Kennedy was. Throughout the '60s, '70s, and '80s it is safe to say she was second only to Queen Elizabeth as being the most famous woman in the world. You saw her image just about every day of your life in magazines, newspapers, books or on the tube. You heard about her on the radio. She was nearly as familiar to you as a member of your own family and it would have been impossible not to have recognized her instantly. And there she was, from the land of the surreal, suddenly walking directly toward me.

Certain moments in your life create such an impact that they remain frozen in time forever in your memory. You replay them over and over in your mind, noticing and renoticing every detail in the mental image. This was such a moment for me.

She wore a loose-fitting burgundy blouse with narrow, vertical, gold stripes and a black skirt cut at the knees. Her hair was the brown, shoulder-length style we were so used to seeing in photographs. In fact, although she was over fifty at the time, Jackie appeared remarkably to have aged not a day since she had been the First Lady of the United States. She looked *exactly* the same.

And she was gorgeous. Drop-dead gorgeous, as the expression goes. Stunningly, exceedingly beautiful. A woman *everyone* would look twice at, even if she weren't already so overwhelmingly famous.

Jackie walked out onto the street in front of my cab and peered inside, trying to see if there was already a passenger in the back seat. If I could have pushed an ejection button and sent my passenger flying off into the stratosphere I would certainly have done so, and Jackie would have gotten in.

But it was not to be. She saw that my taxi was occupied and then spotted another cab, a Checker, without a passenger in it directly next to mine on my left. As she walked around the front of my cab and entered the narrow space between this other cab and my own, I realized that in a moment she would be right next to me and, because my window was already rolled down, I would be able to speak to her. I felt a distinct rush that must have been a release of adrenaline, and then, as the moment arrived with Jackie Kennedy standing beside me, I found that my mouth had opened and words had begun to dribble out of it.

'Hello, Mrs Onassis,' I said sheepishly.

Right away it didn't sound right. Sure, her name was actually 'Jackie Onassis' because she'd married Aristotle Onassis, but it didn't fit her. In my mind, and I think in everybody's mind, she would always be 'Jackie *Kennedy*'. I thought maybe I should have just said, 'Hello, Jackie', but, anyway, it was too late. The words had been said and she'd heard me and now she was putting her attention on me. I feared she might scowl at me or just ignore me entirely, but she didn't – she *smiled* at me.

It was a warm smile that, interestingly, made *me* feel special, as if somehow we had known each other for a long time. It was a smile that communicated that she knew who she was and was quite aware of and caring about how her presence affected other people, and that she had mastered the elements of fame.

But more than that, it was a smile that brought back an era. Here was Camelot, not gone, but returning to life once again. Here was John F. Kennedy and the idealism of my generation. Here was the woman in the pink suit covered with the president's blood, catapulted out of history, standing right next to me, undefeated, triumphant.

Jackie reached forward to open the door of the Checker cab on my left and as she did so I could see through the window that the driver of that cab was an old-time professional, an American, about fifty years old. Here was a guy who could easily be typecast in a commercial or a movie as 'taxi driver'. He had an Archie Bunker kind of appearance.

Jackie Kennedy opened the rear door of his cab and started to get in, but before she could sit down, this driver turned around in his seat and looked right at her – he had something to say. With his face contorted into a snarl, and with a voice that was somewhere between a growl and an outright scream, out came these exact words:

'I'M ONLY GOING UPTOWN!'

'Oh my God,' I said to my passenger, 'I can't believe he spoke to her that way!'

'Oh my God,' she echoed, 'I can't believe it, either!'

But Jackie batted not an eye. She was, in fact, going uptown and stepped into the guy's cab with her companion, completely undisturbed by the driver's incredible lack of manners.

So there he was, the taxi driver of old, himself a vestige of a bygone era. I believe I can safely say that if this guy wasn't going to take Jackie Kennedy *down*town, he wasn't going to take *you* to Brooklyn. But not to worry, today a perfectly nice fellow named Ramesh will drive you to Brooklyn, or to the Bronx for that matter, without a word of protest.

And *that*, ladies and gentlemen, is what's changed in the taxi business in New York City.

Along with one other thing – did someone say 'Checker cab'?

How I brought about the demise of the Checker Motor Company

Now here's something I can't blame on the mayor. In fact, I hate to admit it, but it may have been *my* fault: the Checkers are gone. The beloved Checkers – these were the taxis you see in any movie set in New York City between 1956 and about 1990. Built like tanks, they had extended room in the back, flat floorboards with no uncomfortable 'hump' in the middle, and two folding 'jump seats' that enabled five adults (or twenty midgets) to sit back there. These vehicles have become nostalgia items for anyone who grew up or lived in New York during those years.

Most people don't know that the Checkers were manufactured by the Checker Motor Company, which was not a subsidiary of General Motors or any other conglomerate, but was an independent company on its own. Located in Kalamazoo, Michigan, nearly all the cars that rolled off that assembly line were specifically built to be taxicabs. To make it easier for taxi fleets to replace broken parts and to keep costs down, they stopped redesigning the Checkers in 1956. So the Checkers looked like they were old cars even though they may have been relatively new.

But the Checker Motor Company had big problems. After the gasoline crisis in 1979, many taxi fleet owners switched to Chevrolets, Fords and Dodges. In the highly competitive world of automobile manufacturing, Checker was losing ground and by 1981 was barely treading water.

How was I to know that an innocent conversation between myself and a certain passenger would provide the coup de grâce for these fabulous cars? I'm asking you in advance to please not hate me. Okay, here's the story…

In the second week of July, 1981, I was driving a Checker cab that was owned by my friend Itzy at a garage called West Side Ignition. At West Side Ignition they had a saying: 'If it's not broken, don't fix it. And if it *is* broken, don't fix it.' So when I'd bring the car in for an oil change and mention to Itzy that the shocks were basically gone, Itzy would tell me that as long as the cab was in running condition, to hell with the shocks, just go out and drive. Apparently 'running condition' meant that your condition would be better if you were running instead of trying to drive the damned thing.

Anyway, I was driving this Checker when I was hailed by a middle-aged suburban Workerbee in a business suit who looked like any other commuter on his way home from work. He asked me to bring him to Penn Station, a fifteen-minute trip, and he settled back into his seat and opened up a newspaper. It looked to be an uneventful ride until, about two blocks from where we'd started, the cab ran over a particularly nasty pothole.

Now, the Checkers were strong cars and they had a reputation for being indestructible, but they didn't exactly give you a smooth ride. When we hit the pothole, the cab kind of went KA-BOOM, and I found myself momentarily bouncing up and down on the front seat. In fact, the car had taken the pothole so badly that I felt a need to apologize to my passenger.

'Sorry,' I said with a laugh, 'I guess they don't make them like they used to.' Not that they really made them any differently than they ever did. It was just something to say.

My passenger, who up to this point hadn't said a word to me, suddenly came alive. He put down his newspaper, opened up his briefcase, and took out a notepad and a pen.

'I'd like you to do something for me,' he said. 'I'd like you to tell me everything you *don't* like about Checkers. I'll write down what you say.'

Well, I thought this was fine. Someone wants to know what *I* think. I started in with a vengeance.

'First of all, obviously they can't take bumps worth a damn,' I said. He wrote it down.

'The gas mileage is awful. They only get eight or nine miles per gallon.' He wrote *that* down.

'Lousy acceleration.'

'What else?'

'Squeaky brakes.'

'What else?'

Now I was really getting into it. 'These dashboards are so old-fashioned. They slope straight down so you can't put anything on top of them. You know, they stopped redesigning these cars in 1956.'

He wrote quickly to keep up with me, but if I spoke too fast he would hold me up until he could get it all down. It seemed to be a matter of some concern to him that he recorded every word I said.

'What else?'

'Well, the trunk doesn't spring up when you push the button to open it. There's no place to grip it.'

It was true. Whenever the trunk needed to be opened, the driver had to get out of the cab and pry it open with his fingertips. The privately owned Checkers all had customized handles – installed by the owners themselves, not the Checker Motor Company – on the trunks to overcome this problem.

'Really,' I groaned, 'what kind of a car company makes a car – a taxi, no less – with a trunk that makes it a challenge to open it?'

'Okay, what else?'

'The goddamned battery is back there in the trunk where there's no ventilation. When you start working at a new garage, they give you a big speech on your first day warning you not to hold a cigarette in your hand when you open the trunk because it might set off an explosion if the battery happens to be bad and is giving off fumes! You know, when batteries go bad they emit sulfuric acid, which is flammable. Whoever heard of a battery being in the trunk, anyway? Why don't they put it under the hood like in all other cars?'

It went on like this until we arrived at Penn Station. I told him everything anyone could possibly imagine could be wrong with Checkers, and it felt wonderful.

'So what is this,' I asked, 'some kind of taxi driver therapy?'

'Hell, no,' my passenger said, 'the Chairman of the Board of the Checker Motor Company is an old childhood friend of mine and I'm having lunch with him in Kalamazoo next Wednesday. I'm going to tell him everything you told me.' And with that he handed me the money for the ride along with a generous tip and disappeared into the crowd in Penn Station.

I sat there kind of dumbfounded for a minute in my beat-up cab. Gee, I thought, maybe someday this will result in better Checkers being made. Maybe the Chairman of the Board will be impressed with my astute observations and he'll fix up all the things I said were wrong. Maybe something *I* said will really make a difference! I thought of all the people in America who would be riding around in better cars.

*

Well, it didn't exactly work out that way. Three weeks later I heard on the radio that the Checker Motor Company was going out of business! And, indeed, in July, 1982 the last Checker came off the assembly line.

So here's what must have happened: my passenger did, in fact, have lunch with his old childhood pal the next Wednesday in Kalamazoo. But unbeknownst to my passenger, his old friend was desperately trying to decide at that time whether or not to take out yet another massive loan to keep the company afloat. He tries to put his troubles out of his mind for an hour by having lunch with his childhood buddy whom he hasn't seen in years. He wants to reminisce about the good old days.

But *noooo,* his old pal pulls out this goddamned list of goddamned complaints about his cars that was dictated to him by a real, goddamned New York City taxi driver – as if he doesn't already know what's wrong with his own cars. Later that night, after kicking the cat and screaming at the kids – or maybe kicking the kids and screaming at the cat – he decides *screw it,* it's just not worth the frustration. He's got enough to retire on anyway, so he's going in tomorrow to tell the Board it's all over.

And there went our beloved Checkers.

So you see, it really wasn't *my* fault. If blame is to be placed, it should rest on the shoulders of that guy who was in my cab, not *me.* The trouble was he didn't ask me what I *liked* about Checkers. If he did, I would have told him about the jump seats and the miles of room in the back. I would have told him about the flat floorboards and how, if you were driving a Checker, it would bring you extra business every night because there were always some passengers who would let other types of cabs go by when they saw you coming. In fact, I once missed getting Andy Warhol in my cab because the cab I was driving was *not* a Checker. Although no one was in my cab, a Chevrolet, he let me drive right past him so he could take the Checker that was behind me.

But, alas, history cannot be rewritten. The Checkers are gone. And I do apologize for whatever role I may have played in bringing about this catastrophe.

Don't hate me... *please.*

Come on, don't throw my book in the garbage can. That's not nice. Forgiveness is an important virtue, didn't someone say that once?

Sorry... okay?

4

Celebrities

Certainly one thing that has not changed is a scene such as this: two teenage girls and their mothers, *Agogers* (people who are 'agog') from Georgia on their first trip to New York, piled into my cab at the Waldorf Astoria Hotel on a Saturday evening at 7.30 p.m., en route to the Broadway show *Beauty and the Beast.*

'Hey,' the teenager sitting beside me said as we hit traffic heading into Times Square, 'have you ever had a celebrity in your taxi?'

'Sure,' I replied, 'I've had lots of them.'

'Really?!'

'As a matter of fact,' I said, 'I once had the man who co-wrote the songs of the show you're going to see.'

'Wow, what's his name?'

'Howard Ashman.'

No response. She'd never heard of the late, great lyricist.

'Have you ever had a movie star?'

'Sure.'

'Wow! Really? You *have*? Who? Who?'

'Well, I've had Lauren Bacall.'

No response. Obviously this girl was not a fan of classic cinema.

'How about Leonardo DiCaprio?' I replied, hoping to hit a home run.

'Holy Jesus! Leonardo DiCaprio! In *this* cab?' At which point all four of them began fondling the upholstery, hoping some of Leo's charisma would rub off on them.

What is it about celebrities, anyway? Are they really any different than you and me? Well, in a sense, no. Their food goes in one end and comes out the other, just like everyone else's (although it may start out as sushi from Nobu's for them and a tuna melt from Frank's deli for you and me). But the nature of the lives they are living is really quite different than any other type of person. For example…

Starlight

I was cruising down Columbus Avenue one evening in 1987 when I was hailed at 77th Street by a middle-aged man wearing a tuxedo. He opened the rear door, but instead of getting in, he leaned forward and inspected the condition of the compartment and picked up a couple of errant pieces of paper from the floorboard. Deciding that my taxi now met his high standards, he then asked me to wait a minute while he retrieved his friends from a restaurant on the avenue. One of his friends, he said, was a 'major VIP'.

Well, my curiosity was certainly aroused. Who could this Very Important Person be? In a few moments the man in the tuxedo reappeared from the restaurant with another man, also wearing a tux, and two women in fashionable evening dresses. The cause of all the fuss, it turned out, was this other man. He was Douglas Fairbanks, Jr.

It was a name you would recognize if you were past a certain age. Douglas Fairbanks, Jr, had been a movie star, a leading man, in the 1930s and was the son of Douglas Fairbanks, Sr, himself a big star from the silent movie era. I was familiar with Jr mostly because he was a pitch man for the wool industry and would appear in that capacity in television commercials.

We drove down Columbus Avenue a mere eleven blocks, to

Lincoln Center. As Mr Fairbanks opened the door of my cab and stepped out into the plaza there, he was immediately surrounded by photographers snapping away, their strobe lights creating an explosion of brightness in the cool night air. He posed for the paparazzi, flashing a winning smile and looking altogether dapper. Apparently a special event of some kind was being held that night at Lincoln Center and the media were waiting for the stars to arrive.

After I drove away in anonymity, I had some thoughts about this phenomenon of celebrity. Consider this: although the glow of Douglas Fairbanks, Jr's movie career had faded away nearly *fifty years* prior to that night, he was *still* being treated by the mortals around him with the care and adulation that you and I never receive for even a single day in our lives.

No, they are not the same as the rest of us. There is truly a phenomenon at work here. It's like a force of nature, a type of energy. The physics of mass communications, if you will.

It can be interesting to observe how different celebrities deal with it. Some, like Douglas Fairbanks, Jr, are quite comfortable with it. Others, like John Lennon the two times I saw him on the street, resist it by trying to remain unrecognized behind dark glasses, scarves and various disguises. And then there are those who, like rodeo cowboys riding on the back of a bull, can't seem to get enough of it and will go out of their way to let you know who they are.

Leonardo Di who?

One pleasant Tuesday night in the summer of 1996 I found myself waiting once again in the taxi queue in front of the Bowery Bar in the East Village. The popular Tuesday night party *Beige* was in full swing there and it was a good place to get a fare during an otherwise slow night shift.

I finally got to the front of the line when a group of rowdy kids, probably too young to have been in there in the first place, emerged from the bar, playfully pushing and shoving each other as they approached my cab. Other than the fact that they were loud and goofing around, I noticed three things: 1) one of them was smoking a cigar that was bigger than his face, 2) one of them was a model-gorgeous female and the others were all guys, and 3) there were five of them.

Now there were two problems here. Cigars, of course, are a no-no in a taxicab. And New York City taxis by law are only allowed to carry four passengers. But this group was probably drunk, definitely raucous and they had jumped into my cab so quickly that I decided that playing taxicab cop was too much of an effort and decided to just drive them where they wanted to go without a protest. Three of the guys and the girl crammed themselves onto the back seat and a fellow who must have weighed in excess of three hundred pounds joined me in the front. And off we went.

Our destination was a club called Spy on Greene Street in Soho, a short ride. I opened the windows to allow for some ventilation of the cigar smoke and was being pretty much oblivious to the laughter and clamor surrounding me when a male voice from the back seat suddenly grabbed my attention.

'Hey, driver,' the voice said.

'Yeah?' I called back.

'Hey, you know, this is Leonardo DiCaprio you've got back here!'

'It is?'

'Yeah!'

'Leonardo Di *who*?'

'Leonardo *DiCaprio*!'

'So – who is Leonardo DiCaprio?' I asked. This was before *Titanic* and I'd never heard of him.

A second voice belonging to the blond-haired kid smoking the cigar now joined in the conversation.

'Don't you know who I am?' he cried out.

'Uhhh… nooo…'

'I'm an actor, man!'

'Oh.'

'Did you see *This Boy's Life*?' he asked.

'Oh, I've heard of that movie,' I said, 'but I haven't seen it. You were in that?'

'I played with *De Niro,* man!'

'Wow! Really!'

'How about *What's Eating Gilbert Grape?* Did you see that?'

'No, sorry, I didn't see that one, either. You were in that?'

'Yeah!'

I was certainly out of the loop. I would have liked to have discussed some of his work with him, but I hadn't seen any of the kid's movies.

'Are you in anything that's coming out soon?' I asked.

'Yeah, we just finished *Romeo and Juliet,*' he said.

Well, here was something we could talk about. I know my *Romeo and Juliet* well and a lively conversation ensued between the two of us about this new version.

'Who plays Mercutio?' I wanted to know. 'Who plays Tybalt? It's set in modern times? Really! Hmmm… I wonder if that will work,' and so on.

Our discussion continued until we arrived at Spy. As everyone else piled out of the cab, Leonardo DiWho surprised me. He stayed inside and started asking *me* questions about what it's like to be a taxi driver.

Now, this impressed me – a lot. It brought to mind the difference between *interesting* versus *interested.* I don't think there's anything wrong about trying to be interesting, but I think it's more admirable by far to be interested. For one thing, being interested makes you smarter. You will learn things by being interested. And, in addition to that, being interested gives the people you are talking to the feeling that *they* are important and that you care about them. It bolsters their self-esteem and makes them stronger. In my opinion, simply being interested is one of humanity's most noble virtues. It doesn't have to be a dog eat dog world.

So here was this kid smoking a cigar, a movie star, who you might expect to be the epitome of being *interesting,* instead turning the tables and being *interested.* What a breath of fresh air.

'Who was the biggest celebrity tipper you ever had in your cab?' he asked me.

'Believe it or not, it was John McEnroe,' I replied. 'He gave me double the meter.'

'Well,' Leonardo DiWho said, 'I'm gonna give you *triple* the meter!'

And he did.

I had a feeling this kid was going places and I didn't want to forget his name, so I wrote it down on my trip sheet. My daughter, Suzy, was fourteen at the time and I'd never once been able to impress her by dropping the names of any of the celebrities I've had in my cab. Nevertheless, when I saw Suzy the next day, I told her I had a celebrity in my cab the previous night.

Looking down at my trip sheet, I read the name with some difficulty.

'Have you ever heard of this guy… Leonardo… Di… uh… Cap…rio?'

A shriek came out of the mouth of my daughter that nearly shattered the wine glasses in the cabinet. This was followed by moans of the deepest anguish when it was learned that I had failed to obtain his autograph, a sin for which I have never been forgiven.

Oh, yes. *She* knew who he was.

Another question I'm frequently asked is, 'How many celebrities have you had in your cab?' I've wondered about this myself, so I made a list of every celebrity, big or small, I could think of who'd ever climbed into the back seat. By 'big' I mean a major star, like Leonardo DiCaprio. 'Small' would be someone who is known only locally, like a radio DJ or broadcast news personality.

The grand total, as of this writing, is 114. Some of these celebrities I've had more than once (Dick Clark – three times!), so if I counted each time *that* happened the total would be 122. And if I were able to count the ones I didn't recognize, I'm sure the number would be God knows how many. But however you look at it, it's a lot of celebs. So many, in fact, that it lends itself to categorization. Here are some of the stand outs:

Movie Stars – 17 – Lauren Bacall, Sean Penn, Dennis Hopper, Jane Seymour, Richard Dreyfuss, Robin Williams, Matt Dillon, Dan Aykroyd, Eli Wallach, Kevin Kline, Bill Pullman, Diane Keaton, Carroll O'Connor, Kevin Bacon, Tom Hulce, Douglas Fairbanks, Jr and, of course, Leo.

Pop Music Stars – 9 – Ray Davies (The Kinks), Johnny Rzeznik (Goo Goo Dolls), Paul Simon, Art Garfunkel, Carly Simon, Diahann Carroll, Gregg Allman, Derek Trucks, James Taylor.

Crooners – 3 – Tony Bennett, Frank Sinatra, Jr, Eddie Fisher.

Folk Singers – 3 – Peter Yarrow (Peter, Paul and Mary), Suzanne Vega, Richie Havens.

Famous Writers – 5 – Norman Mailer, Jimmy Breslin, Harrison Salisbury, Rex Reed, Liz Smith.

Offspring of Celebrities Who Are Celebrities Themselves – 4 – Caroline Kennedy, Lucie Arnez, Douglas Fairbanks, Jr, Steven Mailer (son of Norman).

Talk Show Hosts – 3 – Dick Cavett, David Susskind, Tom Snyder.

Band Leaders of Late-Night Talk Shows – 2 – Paul Schaeffer (Letterman), Max Weinberg (Conan O'Brian).

Big-Time Businessmen Who Named Their Companies After Themselves – 2 – Leon Hess (Hess Oil and owner of the NY Jets football team), Frank ('it takes a tough man to make a tender chicken') Purdue. *Writers of Famous Christmas Songs* – 2 – Mel Tormé ('The Christmas Song', aka 'Chestnuts Roasting on an Open Fire'), J. Fred Coots ('Santa Claus is Coming to Town').

Porn Stars – 3 – Hyapatia Lee, Sharon Mitchell, Cara Lott.

Mick Jagger Exes – 2 – Marianne Faithfull, Bianca Jagger.

Fugitive Hippies – 1 – Abbie Hoffman.

That's right. I had a famous fugitive hippie in my cab, and there aren't too many of those around. Or perhaps I should say a 'former' fugitive hippie…

Abbie Hoffman

I was cruising up 8th Avenue one night in February, 1982, when I was hailed by two men on the street. One was a normal-looking, forty-something fellow and the other turned out to be a dark-haired, raving motormouth who spoke to his traveling companion in a semi-hysterical rant without giving him a chance to get a word in edgewise. We continued up 8th Avenue to Central Park West until we reached 65th Street, where the man with the obsessive outflow got out of the cab, leaving the other passenger with me. I turned right onto transverse and we proceeded across the park to the East Side.

'That was Abbie Hoffman,' the man said. 'I'm his parole officer.'

Abbie Hoffman, if you're too young to remember him, was an iconic counter-culture figure from the '60s. He founded the Youth International Party (the "Yippies") and received vast amounts of publicity by engineering stunts and demonstrations which mocked some of the dubious values of American society. He had been convicted of dealing cocaine in 1973 and became a fugitive until 1980, when he re-emerged and served a brief prison term.

It was a surprise and something of a revelation to be able to be a 'fly on the wall' during this ride. A surprise because Abbie Hoffman had seemed to me to be something of a folk legend, more like a Johnny Appleseed or a Paul Bunyon than a real person. Yet there he was.

And a revelation to observe the condition he was actually in. I was saddened but not altogether surprised several years later to learn that he had committed suicide.

However, it is another iconic personage from the '60s (and beyond) who is the answer to this frequently asked question: 'Of all the celebrities you've had in your cab, which one is your favorite?'

Paul Simon's warmth

On two occasions I have been honored to transport the derriere of the great Paul Simon in my taxicab. The composer of 'Bridge Over Troubled Water', 'Mrs, Robinson', 'The Boxer' and so many other wonderful songs, Paul Simon is someone who I can truly say has enriched my life through his music. It can be a little overwhelming, however, to meet someone in person whom you have admired for so long. What do you say to a living legend? What, when you find yourself suddenly face to face with such a larger-than-life character, do you talk about?

Why, baseball, of course.

I was heading uptown on Central Park West on a lovely day in June, 1983, looking for my next passenger, when I spotted him standing there with a doorman on the opposite side of the street. They both had an 'I want a cab' expression on their faces which I took as my cue to make one of those sweeping U-turns that taxis in New York City are famous for. Taking care not to run over my favorite songwriter and thus bring to an end the long series of Simon and Garfunkel reunions, I pulled my cab around to where they were standing, and Paul got in.

He wanted to go to the East Side, so we headed through Central Park in that direction. I noticed Paul was wearing an unusual baseball cap with an insignia on it that I didn't recognize so, seeking an entrance point from which to start a conversation, I asked him what his hat was all about. He told me it was a hat from a Japanese baseball team, that he'd 'played a stadium over there', and that the hat was a souvenir. I asked him jokingly which position he had played and, matching the spirit of my question, Paul replied that he'd played 'guitar'.

I noticed that we had found some common ground upon which to communicate and that there was some rapport between us, so I decided to steer the discussion to an area of fertile soil when baseball is the subject of conversation in New York – the Yankees. I had heard or read somewhere that Paul was a Yankee fan, which might be expected of the person who wrote the line, 'Where have you gone, Joe DiMaggio?', and I was not wrong.

As our chat about the Yankees got going, I could see that Paul was emotionally involved with the franchise and its meaning to New York. He spoke knowledgeably about the players and the problems the organization was having. And he had nothing positive to say about George Steinbrenner, the owner of the team, or Billy Martin, who was in one of his many incarnations as the Yankee manager at the time, even going so far as saying that the two of them were not only bad for baseball, but bad for New York City as well.

I was quite impressed by the passion with which he spoke. It was obvious that baseball in general and the Yankees in particular were things that were important to him. So involved had Paul become in our discussion of the subject, in fact, that he stayed on in my cab for a minute after we reached his destination in order to wrap up the conversation – a great honor, from my point of view. Once he finally did leave I was left with the impression that in Paul's world the travails of Julio down by the schoolyard and Cecilia up in his bedroom were of no more importance than the slings and arrows of Willie Randolph at second and Dave Winfield in right.

The memory of our conversation stayed with me for some time. I found myself wondering, whenever George or Billy would make the news with some new blunder, what Paul would have said about it. He had become for me the conscience of the Yankees. And then one day, out of nowhere, an idea hit me with the impact of a Goose Gossage fastball: *Paul Simon would make the perfect owner of the New York Yankees.* A native New Yorker, a lifelong Yankee fan, an important contributor to the legacy of the team through his music, a caring, intelligent and disciplined person, and the possessor of some serious wealth – somehow it all just fit. Yes! Paul Simon, the one man who could rescue our Yankees from the tyranny of the wicked King George. I decided that if fate ever put Paul back in my cab, I would do my best to sell him on the idea.

As it turned out, fate was kind.

On an unusually frigid day in late November, 1984 – just a few weeks after the conclusion of yet another dismal baseball season for the Yankees – I again spotted Paul standing with his doorman at the same building on Central Park West. Once again I made an outrageous turn to get to him and, after refreshing his memory about our previous conversation, I wasted no time in getting to the matter at hand. I told him I had an idea that he'd probably think was crazy at first, but I wanted him to at least take a look at it. And then I laid it on him.

'I want you to buy the Yankees,' I said.

It certainly took him by surprise.

'*Me*? You want *me* to buy the *Yankees*?' he said incredulously.

I told him it wasn't as crazy as it sounds. A lot of things happen that seem bizarre until we get used to them. I told him he had some pretty good qualifications, having written that line about Joe DiMaggio, and being a native New Yorker, and all. I could see he was softening up on the idea. He started tossing the concept around in his mind. But he hit a snag right away.

'I don't have *that* kind of money,' he said. 'You should talk to McCartney.'

I took this as a minor stumbling block that any salesman would encounter en route to closing a deal. All I had to do was show my client that where there's a will there's a way. I asked him what he thought the team was worth. After giving it some thought he guessed that ninety or a hundred million dollars would do the trick. Arriving at this figure, however, was not something that helped my cause. But then I realized that what he'd given me was in sales parlance just an 'illegitimate excuse'. Now it was my job to strip away all the illegitimate excuses until we came to what the real objection was, if, in fact, there was one. So I suggested setting up a consortium of investors with Paul as the principal owner.

'What about Billy Joel?' I asked.

'Oh, yeah, he's a *big* Yankee fan!' Paul replied with genuine enthusiasm.

Now we were getting somewhere – the seed had been planted and was starting to grow. I could see in my mind the same image that I was sure was in Paul's: a large conference room in Yankee Stadium, Paul sitting at the head of the table, Billy Joel at his side, and about twenty seats filled with rock singers and movie stars. A big decision had to be made: *should Tommy John be offered a new contract even though he's forty-one years old?*

But Paul raised a new objection. He began talking, quite

sincerely, about his basic purpose line. He'd always wanted to be a rock singer, he said, and that's what he had dedicated himself to and had become. He told me that there had been times when he had considered doing things that would have been divergences from his purpose line, but they never came to anything, and that his steadfastness to his purpose was one of the reasons for his success. Although owning the Yankees sounded intriguing, it would ultimately be something that would take him away from his work.

As a salesman I had to consider this statement, convincing as it might sound, as just another illegitimate excuse and I went to work at chopping it down. My objective was to show Paul how owning the Yankees would actually enhance his basic purpose. I pointed out that buying the franchise would give him access to Yankee Stadium as a concert arena. He could book concerts, including himself as a solo artist and himself with Garfunkel, on dates when the Yankees were unlikely to draw large crowds. This concept seemed to sit well with him as he immediately started looking at what might stand in the way of his acquiring the team.

'I don't think George would ever sell,' he said.

Now here, I had to admit, we had a formidable, perhaps even insurmountable, obstacle. What if it wasn't a matter of money? What if the team simply wasn't for sale at any price? It seemed that the only possibility of overcoming this barrier would be to solve the mystery of what it is that makes George tick. We went to work at it.

Why, we wondered, would George Steinbrenner want to be the owner of a baseball team, anyway? Was it because he loved baseball? Possibly, but we didn't think so. Was it for the money? Again, this was possible but, knowing as much as we've all come to know about George, it didn't seem to ring true that money would be his real motivation. What was concluded, after some discussion, was that George is a person who needs recognition and approval in a big way.

Now there could be various ways of achieving recognition and approval. Certainly one way was to become famous and loved as the owner of a baseball team. But there could be other ways, too… like performing in front of thousands of people and singing lively songs while a band plays behind you.

So there it was, the solution to the problem! Paul would put together a group of investors, the matter of the money would be resolved, and everyone would get what they want: Paul – the Yankees. George – well, first George will get training for his new career. Voice control, stage presence, a new wardrobe. And then, before you know it, the world will be enamored of, astonished by and delirious for the harmonies created by George and his new partner.

The group will be called *Simon and Steinbrenner*. Sorry, Art.

We had arrived at Paul's destination, the Brill Building on Broadway and 49th. There was still one detail he had some attention on – the matter of contacting George, conducting the negotiations and closing the sale. It was something he didn't particularly want to get involved in until it was really necessary. So Paul decided to offer me a deal.

'Tell you what,' he said as he started to step out of my cab into the freezing afternoon air, 'if you can get George to sign the papers, I'll give you a percentage.'

And with that he smiled, waved goodbye, and went on his way.

I drove less than a block down Broadway, already doing the math in my head of what a percentage would bring me, when my next passenger, a middle-aged woman, hailed me from the frozen street and jumped in. She sat in the same spot in back where Paul Simon had just been sitting.

'Hey, you know who I just had in my cab?' I said to her… 'Paul

Simon!'

'You *did?*' she said in amazement. She then started moving her body back and forth against the seat. *'You mean I'm sitting in Paul Simon's warmth?!'*

A Woody Allen story

Of all the celebrities in New York, I don't think there is any who is as much identified with the city nor as visible in the city as Woody Allen. I have often seen him around town – going into Knicks games at Madison Square Garden, directing or acting in his own movies on the street, or just walking around. It's easy to spot him. He looks exactly the same in real life as he does on the screen.

He has also always been the most locatable celebrity in New York City. You always knew where this guy would be on a Monday night – at Michael's Pub on 55th Street between 2nd and 3rd Avenues. For many years Woody played the clarinet in a Dixieland band there without ever missing a date. He was *always* there on Monday nights.

In 1977, for example, when the Academy Awards ceremonies were still being held on Mondays, Woody's movie *Annie Hall* won Oscars for Best Director, Best Original Screenplay and Best Picture. Was Woody in Hollywood to pick up his Oscar? No, he was playing the clarinet at Michael's Pub.

It so happens that Michael's Pub, before it moved in 1996, was situated on the ground floor of a high-rise office building that is occupied almost entirely by lawyers. Many of them work late so this building is an excellent place to look for a fare between the hours of seven and ten on any weeknight. If a taxi driver waits there for a few minutes between these hours, he will be sure to get a customer. Therefore I would often be there, and if it was a Monday night I'd always wonder if I would be seeing Woody Allen.

At 9.25 p.m. he would come out of the place. It was that predictable. Sometimes he'd be alone, sometimes he'd be with Soon-Yi, sometimes with his father. He had a Mercedes and a driver waiting for him. If people gathered around him and asked him to pose for a photograph, he would oblige for a minute and then his driver, in what appeared to be a rehearsed drill, would wrench him away and usher him into his car. I saw this many times and I always considered it to be a treat, one of those special, little New York experiences. And there was an additional treat from a business point of view. The people who had come to Michael's Pub to see Woody Allen would also become taxi customers, so adding them onto the lawyers made Monday nights even better over there. For some reason nearly all of them were Europeans, usually from France, Denmark, Sweden, Germany or Holland. I supposed that Woody was big in those countries and apparently it was well known that you could see him in person at this particular location. Perhaps it was even better known over there than it was here, because my passengers were rarely Americans.

One Monday night in October, 1992 I was waiting there on 55th Street when the first people started to emerge from Michael's. Two French women got into my taxi who were taking a short trip down to the Waldorf Astoria Hotel on 49th and Lex, a three-minute ride.

'How did you like Woody Allen?' I asked.

'Oh,' one of them said in a pleasing accent, 'he was so wonderful!'

'He looks just the same as he does in the movies!' the other one chimed in.

'He does, doesn't he?' I agreed.

It was a conversation I'd had many times. I never got tired of hearing people's reactions to having just seen Woody Allen. It was, as noted, a treat.

As my passengers left my cab, I realized I could probably zip back up to 55th and catch another fare coming out of the place, since it usually took about ten minutes for all the people to leave. So I made a left on 48th Street, another left on 3rd Avenue, and in three minutes I was once again sitting in front of Michael's Pub. A middle-aged couple from Germany immediately entered my cab who wanted to go to the Marriott Marquis Hotel in Times Square.

'How did you like Woody Allen?' I asked.

I watched for their reaction in the mirror. But instead of the enthusiastic response I expected, they looked at each other in confusion, obviously wondering why I would ask them such a question.

'Uh,' the gentleman said with a trace of apology in his voice, 'we, uh, we don't much care for Woody Allen.'

I was startled. No one had ever said anything like this before.

'Weren't you just coming from Michael's Pub?' I asked.

'Yes.'

'Didn't you see Woody Allen?' I asked, knowing for sure that he had indeed been there because the French women had just told me that they'd seen him.

'Oh, no,' the man from Germany said, 'we didn't go to see Woody Allen. We went to see the Dixieland band.'

'*What*? You didn't know that Woody Allen is *in* that band?' I asked incredulously. 'He plays the clarinet!'

They looked at each other as if I was completely out of my mind.

'Woody Allen?… clarinet?' the man responded softly, trying

without success to link these two apparently incongruous items in his mind.

'Yes! He plays in the Dixieland band there every Monday night!' I replied with a touch of desperation in my voice. 'He's *always* there!'

My exclamation received no response. I could tell from their silence that they were trying to figure out if there was even the slightest chance that what I was telling them was the truth or if, more likely, their cab driver had been discharged prematurely from a mental institution. Some salesmanship was going to be necessary.

'Really,' I continued, 'it's very well known – he's *always* there on a Monday night!'

'Uh, why would Woody Allen want to be in a Dixieland band?' the man asked cautiously.

'I don't know,' I replied. 'Maybe it relaxes him.'

'But he must be too busy with his movies to be in a band,' he said.

'Yeah, you would think so, but he's there every Monday night. I see him all the time.'

'You do?'

'Yes, really!'

After a couple of minutes of basically just insisting that Woody Allen playing the clarinet was a reality, I could see that I was beginning to win them over. Finally I told them about the French women.

'In fact,' I said, 'I just had two women from France in my cab who'd been in there with you in Michael's Pub. Just five minutes ago! I took them to the Waldorf Astoria Hotel and then I came right back here. And they told me that, yes, Woody Allen was there tonight playing the clarinet. So he was definitely there.'

They looked at each other with expressions on their faces as if to say, 'Well, if the women from France say so it must be true.'

'I *told* you the clarinet player was good,' the German woman said, finally voicing an opinion.

A big smile came over the gentleman's face.

'Wow,' he said, 'I can't wait to tell our son that we saw Woody Allen!'

5

Extreme behavior

Anyone who has been to New York for even a short amount of time knows that one of the characteristics of the city is that there are some really strange people here. They come in three types:

1. *Type One* – people who look strange but act normal. Like the fellow I once had in my cab whose face was totally covered with tattoos yet carried on a perfectly mundane conversation with a female companion all the way to Queens.

2. *Type Two* – people who look strange and also act strange. Like the non-passable cross-dresser who tried to climb over the back seat to get into the front with me and could only be dissuaded by my telling him that I knew he was a man.

3. *Type Three* – people who look normal but act strange. Like the guy who didn't say a word to me in regular speech but instead *sang* to me, Luther Vandross style, for the entirety of the ride.

Consider this: every really strange person who's ever walked the sidewalks of New York gets into a taxicab sooner or later. And some of these people are given over to *extreme behavior.* Which means they must be *dealt with* by the driver…

Screamer

Generally speaking, it is the Type Three – the one who looks perfectly normal - who gives you the most trouble, and a man I picked up one night in April, 1997, was a Type Three indeed. He was about forty years old – average height and weight, nothing unusual about his appearance – so when he got in my cab on 8th Avenue and 44th Street and told me he wanted to go way uptown to Washington Heights, a six-mile trip, I thought nothing of it and just started driving in the direction of the Henry Hudson Parkway, the fastest way to get there.

We drove the first ten blocks in silence. And then, with no provocation whatsoever, the guy just started *screaming* – a low-pitched groan of *aaaaaaaaaahhhhhhhhhhh* – for about five seconds, and then he stopped and sat there with a blank expression on his face as if there was nothing unusual about what he'd just done.

It got my attention.

'What's the matter?' I asked (of course).

He just moved his eyes from one side of the cab to the other and said nothing for a few moments, and then, almost imperceptibly, the word 'sorry' came dribbling out of his mouth.

Oh, boy, the guy was a nut job. Whether or not he was a dangerous nut job or a not-dangerous nut job I did not yet know, but *le job nut* he definitely was. I drove on, not being sure how to handle this particle.

I made a left on 57th Street and caught a red light at 9th Avenue. We sat in silence for thirty seconds, the light turned green, and I started to accelerate. And then, again, a little louder:

aaaaaaaaaaahhhhhhhhhhh!

What the *hell* was the matter with this guy? I pulled over to the curb and stopped the cab.

'What's going *on?*' I asked, the tone of my voice leaning toward hostility.

Once again my passenger examined the interior of the cab and sheepishly apologized for his truly odd behavior.

'You okay?'

'Yes… sorry…'

I looked at him in the mirror and remained confused. He seemed all right even though, clearly, he wasn't all right. Still, since I wasn't sensing any threat to myself, it didn't seem like the right thing to do to just throw him out of the cab. I decided to give him another chance.

'Okay,' I said, 'no more screaming… okay?'

'Yeah, sorry.'

'Do that again and I'm gonna throw you out of my cab,' I said. 'I can't drive like that.'

'Okay, sorry.'

Having laid down the law, I pulled back out onto 57th Street and then caught another red at 10th Avenue. Screamer, as I now thought of him, remained calm and silent. Apparently my scolding had been what was needed to put this guy back in control of his bizarre impulses.

I continued driving straight on 57th Street and in another minute we were zipping up the Henry Hudson Parkway at sixty miles per hour. We passed the 79th Street exit of the parkway, we passed the 96th Street exit, and then:

aaaaaaaaaahhhhhhhhhhh…

It was a bit louder than before, and it was continuous. Apparently my passenger realized I couldn't stop on the parkway and this meant to him that he had been given a free pass to wake up the world. I made what seemed to me to be a strong statement of protest – something along the lines of 'What the fuck is your *problem*?' – but it made no effect and the screaming continued steadily all the way to the Washington Heights exit and ceased the moment we were back on the streets.

I drove the remaining four blocks of the ride in what may have been one of the most uncomfortable silences in the history of taxi driving. Then, as we arrived at his building, Screamer had one more surprise for me. He committed a taxi *faux pas* by opening the right-side, rear door before paying the fare. Being that he'd already demonstrated that he was out of his mind, I jumped on it immediately.

'Pay what's on the meter before you leave the taxi,' I said bluntly.

He glanced in my general direction without making eye contact and started moving out of the cab, as if I hadn't said anything at all.

'If you walk away without paying me we're gonna have a problem,' I declared in what was intended to be a threatening tone, but it was to no avail. He slid out of the opened door and closed it from the street. I was about to jump out of the cab and run after him if he took two steps in the wrong direction, but he didn't try to walk away. Instead he came up to the passenger-side window, which was opened, and expressed his resentment in his own unique way.

He started throwing money at me through the window.

'I never stiffed anyone in my life!' he snarled as singles, fives and a ten or two came flying in my direction. He then marched off in a huff to return to whatever universe he had come from.

I counted the money. Not only had he paid the fare, the guy had given me a $43 tip. A nice bit of change, but when I thought about what he'd put me through, I figured I'd earned it. The stress of that ride… well, I'll tell you – it was enough to make *me* want to scream!

Now I don't want to give you the impression that I hold a grudge of some kind against strange people. To the contrary, oddballs are one of the things that give New York its charm. I mean, with thousands of people who look pretty much the same as each other walking along on the sidewalk, isn't it nice every once in a while to see someone who's dressed up like a Viking? Or a chicken?

Actually, I wish all the truly bizarre people would be that obvious. At least you'd know right away what you're dealing with. But, as we've seen with Screamer, it's the person who appears to be ordinary yet turns out to be really weird – the Type Three – that's likely to be the most trouble. Like the woman who hailed me at the corner of 37th and Lex one evening…

'Just drive'

She was a blonde, youthful and attractive, who climbed into the back seat at about 9 p.m. on a Tuesday in August, 1982. People usually tell me their destination immediately upon entering the cab, but sometimes their attention is so dispersed by something that's going on at that moment that there's a brief time lapse before they realize they have to tell the driver where the hell it is that they want to go. So I normally just pull out into traffic and start driving even if I haven't been supplied with this rather important piece of information.

Which is what I did. But after we'd driven a block and I still didn't know her destination, I thought it was time to make an inquiry.

'So where are you going?' I asked, looking at her in the mirror.

'Just drive,' she replied kind of offhandedly.

Okay, I thought, she must still be in the process of figuring out where she wanted to go. Maybe she knew it was a certain restaurant or a club but she needed to dig the address out of her purse or something. She would probably tell me the street in just a little bit and I supposed we were already heading in the right direction (downtown), so I kept driving straight down Lexington Avenue.

Lex ends at 21st Street, which is a one-way street running west.

So, since I didn't know if she wanted to head east or west, when we got to 25th Street and I still hadn't heard from her, I decided it was time to repeat the question.

'Uh, miss, you still haven't told me where you want to go,' I said politely. 'Where are we going?'

'Just drive,' she said.

Uh-oh. She had appeared on my radar screen as potential trouble. But maybe not.

'Just *drive?*' I asked.

'Just drive,' she repeated.

'You mean you don't care where I go?'

'Just drive.'

I looked at her in the mirror. She wasn't rummaging through her pocketbook trying to find an address – she was gazing out the window. Apparently she really didn't care where I drove. She just wanted to go for a ride.

Well, this was a first. I felt a sense of freedom in that the driver–passenger relationship had been altered in my favor. It was *I* who was now deciding where we would go. This was a new experience, and it felt good.

I made a left on 23rd Street, got a green light at 3rd Avenue and then caught a red at 2nd. I looked at her again in the mirror. Her face was expressionless. She was still looking through her window but it was hard to tell if she was actually seeing whatever was out there or if she was just lost in her own thoughts. What was the story with this person? I liked what she was doing, but it was weird.

I drove to 1st Avenue and stopped briefly at the intersection for a red light and made the left when it turned green. I was now heading uptown, in the opposite direction from which we'd started the ride. It was a moment of truth. I still hadn't been convinced that she *really* didn't care where we drove. I thought maybe if I changed directions it would call her bluff, if she was bluffing, and she would tell me to turn around and head back downtown because, in fact, she really *did* have a destination and that destination would be downtown, because that's where we were going when we'd started the ride.

But she wasn't bluffing. She continued to just gaze out the window.

'Oh my God,' I thought, 'this chick really doesn't care where I go.'

The apprehension I'd felt initially was now gone. This was like a Christmas present. After considering the situation for a moment, I decided to do what any self-respecting New York cabbie would do under these circumstances.

I headed for the highway.

'I'm gonna get on the Drive,' I called back to her, referring to the FDR Drive, the parkway that runs along the east side of Manhattan. It is here where you can drive the fastest, and fast driving is what makes the meter click most frequently. It was a gutsy call, and I wasn't sure she'd go for it. But her response was still more good news.

'Could you turn on the radio, please?' she replied.

Now, when a passenger asks you to turn on the radio, it means they either want to listen to some music or they actually just don't want to talk to you. I didn't care if it was one or the other. The important thing was that this was the final confirmation I needed to know for sure that I had been given the green light, if you will, to aimlessly wander the streets of New York City and get paid for it.

I turned the radio dial to a soft rock station and made a right at 34th Street. Within half a minute we were on the FDR, heading north, and, as I brought the cab up to sixty miles per hour and watched the clicking of the meter reflect the speed at which we were moving, I found that a wide smile had planted itself on my face. Yes sir, I had entered taxi driver heaven!

Surely, I thought, this was as good as it gets. What could be better than this? A passenger gets in your cab and you drive wherever the hell you want and your dearest friend, the meter, just keeps clicking, clicking, *clicking!* Oh, yeah! Oh, *yeah!*

We zipped past the 42nd Street exit. Click. We zoomed past the 96th Street exit. Click-click. 125th Street – clickety-click-click-*click!* But then, as we approached the 155th Street exit, it occurred to me.

This is too good to be true.

Having been thoroughly indoctrinated in the school of 'there's always a catch', I felt a little fizzle waving at me from the bottom of my balloon. Why, I wondered, would anyone do what this young lady was doing?

I looked at her carefully in the mirror. She was still gazing out the window without expression, a sphinx. I began to consider the possibilities:

– something terrible was happening at her apartment and she needed to get away. Maybe she'd had a fight with her boyfriend or husband and was deciding whether or not to break up with him.

– then again, maybe something great had happened. Maybe she'd just won the lottery and was figuring out which friends and relatives were going to get some of the money and which ones would be left out.

– or maybe she was one of those females that do things on totally crazy impulses and she'd just decided as she left her building that what she really needed was 'a ride'.

Hell, I didn't know.

*

I took the FDR as far as it would go and got off at the Dyckman Street exit. I was doing just fine where the meter was concerned, but, oddly enough, I found that I was no longer as interested in running it up as I was in solving the riddle of *her*. My curiosity had gotten the best of me and I began to wonder how I might be able to get the story out of her.

Maybe some small talk would open a crack in the door. We were then in the Inwood section of Manhattan, an area where, for some reason, there's always been an excess of double-parked cars. I took a stab at it.

'It's incredible how many people double-park their cars up here,' I said. 'It's like it's a way of life or something.'

I looked at her in the mirror. Nothing. She continued gazing out her window as if I hadn't said a word. I tried again.

'What are you supposed to do if your car is parked next to the curb and some other car has you boxed in? Sit there and wait for the owner of the double-parked car to show up?'

She had built an invisible wall around herself that was impenetrable to my voice. I decided that my original idea of squeezing every dime out of this ride that I could wasn't such a bad idea after all and drove west on Dyckman about ten blocks to the southbound entrance of the Henry Hudson Parkway, the highway that runs along the west side of Manhattan. And as I picked up speed, my meter was purring again.

We breezed down the Henry Hudson without traffic and came to a stop at a red light at 56th Street, where the parkway ends. It was there that a new thought occurred to me. Jesus, what if she's suicidal? Maybe she's going to pull a gun out of her bag and blow her brains out. Maybe this was 'the last ride'. Given the circumstances, it didn't seem so far-fetched. I studied her again in the mirror. It seemed to me now that the far-away look in her eyes was a mask she wore to obstruct a deep sadness she was feeling.

It wasn't difficult to imagine her going somewhere and overdosing on pills or jumping off a bridge. I felt a desire to help her if I could, but I couldn't think of any way to reach her. Nevertheless, when I got to a red light at 42nd Street, I did my best.

'Uh, miss,' I blurted out, 'are you having some kind of trouble? Do you need someone to talk to?' I thought it was a rather valiant thing to do and felt good about myself for having said something. But I already knew inside what her reply would be.

'Please,' she said, not unkindly, 'just drive.'

Humph. All right, I tried. At least, if I found myself reading about her in the paper the next day, I could live with my conscience. My job isn't crisis intervention. It's Point A to Point B. That's all.

I drove on, but now I wasn't feeling as magnanimous as I had before. In fact, as we approached the next red light at 23rd Street, a new thought crept into my mind. What if this weirdo had no intention of paying me at all? What if she thought she could just ride around Manhattan in a cab all night if she felt like it and then give the driver the slip? Some of these women think all men are suckers and some kind of chauvinistic code protects them from retaliation. What if she was one of those?

Once again I looked at her in the mirror. Suddenly it wasn't hard to imagine her stealing cosmetics in a department store. I decided to do something that would be insulting to any honest passenger, but it's something a cab driver can do if he has serious suspicions that he's not going to be paid. He can ask the passenger to show him the money. Not pay in advance. Just show the money to ascertain that it's there. Given how completely unorthodox this ride had already been, it didn't seem inappropriate to me to ask her to do this. I started thinking about how exactly I was going to say this to her without totally offending her.

But before I could open my mouth, she beat me to the punch by saying these words:

'Please,' she said, 'take me back to where you picked me up.'

Oh. Well, that changed everything. There's no point in asking someone to show you her money when the ride is about to end. They'll either have it or they won't. So I made my next left and headed uptown, back to 37th and Lex, and as I drove I was thinking that if she tried something cute like telling me she had to go inside to get her money, I would lock the doors and drive her to a police precinct. I wasn't going to let myself be made a fool of by this chick. Not after driving her around the city for nearly an hour.

As we pulled up to the same spot where I'd picked her up, the moment of truth was at hand, and the moment of truth turned out to be brief and unspectacular. She handed me the money for the fare along with an average tip, opened the door, and left without saying a word.

I watched her walk down 37th Street and disappear into an apartment building. And at the moment she was gone from my sight, I had a realization. I knew that I would be wondering for the rest of my life just what the hell was going on with that woman. And that I would never know.

And I have been. And I don't.

The hooker reconnaissance unit

In the pre-Giuliani days of wilder-than-it-is-now New York, hookers could be seen hard at work on certain streets in the city and, inevitably, a taxi driver would occasionally get one in his cab as a passenger. Whenever this happened, I looked at it as a break from the usual humdrum and would expect some kind of memorable ride. Rarely was I disappointed.

Now the question could be asked where in my three categories of strange people a hooker should be placed. Is a street hooker someone who looks strange but acts normal? Someone who looks strange and also acts strange? Or someone who looks normal but acts strange? Hmmmm…

Well, I guess it can't be someone who looks normal because, yes, they may look normal for hookers but a girl wearing half a bra, a thong, six-inch heels and nothing else just can't be said to look normal. Sexy, maybe, but not normal. So I guess I'd have to describe a street hooker as someone who looks strange but acts normal. I mean, normal as a passenger. Even though her outfit says 'hooker' in neon lights, she still just wants you to take her somewhere.

Except for the time I had a hooker who looked normal, then acted strange, then looked strange, and then acted normal.

*

Back in the late '70s and into the '80s, there were actually two distinct types of prostitutes walking the pavement in Manhattan. There were the ones who were barely dressed and could mostly be found on the West Side in the vicinity of 11th Avenue between 24th and 45th Streets, and then there were the Central Park South hookers. These ladies dressed conservatively and couldn't be recognized as hookers except by a trained eye because they looked like regular women. Their modus operandi was to approach businessmen as they were about to enter top hotels like the Plaza, the Park Lane, the Ritz or the Essex House and strike a deal right there on the street. They would then enter the hotels with their newly acquired johns as if they were wives or business associates.

One night around midnight a woman in stylish clothing jumped in at Central Park South and 6th Avenue and directed me to drive her down to 11th Avenue and 28th Street. I was heading toward 11th on 57th when unusual back and forth movement in the rear caught my attention. I looked in the mirror and found that one of my male taxi driver fantasies had come true – my passenger was changing her clothes in the back seat, a transformation of Samantha Jones into Samantha Slut. Her designer top and skirt had disappeared, presumably into her bag, and what was now sitting there was a half-naked ho in a see-through teddy, red panties, fishnet stockings and a garter belt.

'It's all over at the hotels,' she complained, as she applied more lipstick and changed her earrings. 'Gotta go where the business at!'

Which was 11th Avenue and 28th Street. The rest of the ride was relatively normal taxi chit-chat until we arrived at that destination, she paid the fare with an above-average tip, and then got out to ply her trade, not that much unlike any other business person.

*

But by the time the mid-'90s rolled around times had changed for the hookers. The mayor was relentless in commanding his police force to rid the streets of its trollops, which meant the heat was always on. The Central Park South hookers were gone and the West Side cruising area was no longer the friendly red-light district it had once been.

Nevertheless, there were still some diehards who were not about to let the world's oldest profession disappear without a fight. One of them hailed me from the corner of 23rd Street and 10th Avenue at 2 a.m. in June, 1997.

She was a small white girl with platinum-blonde hair, wearing a halter top and skin-tight short-shorts with a camel toe, maybe nineteen or twenty years old. Based on her appearance, I made a quick determination that I was about to be dealing with a naïve runaway, someone who had fled from a lousy family situation in Ohio and was now being manipulated by the evil father-figure known as a pimp. The thought crossed my mind that this could be my Travis Bickle moment, that I might be able to help her see the light and go back to Ma and Pa on the farm.

But, as is normally the case when my imagination puts me in the role of white knight on a steed, I was completely wrong. She was anything but a confused little waif.

'Could you take me to 20th and 8th, please?' she asked with a voice that was reminiscent of the sound made by a receptionist in a busy office building. I turned the cab to the east and in a couple of minutes we were on 20th Street, approaching the intersection she desired.

'Go straight toward 7th,' she said.

I did as directed. Looking at her in the mirror, I could see that she was searching for something on the street.

'A little slower, please.'

I brought the cab down to a crawl. She continued to scrutinize the area in the middle of the block until she suddenly seemed satisfied that whatever she'd wanted to see had been seen.

'Okay,' she said with an upbeat expression on her face, 'take me back to where you picked me up.' I made a right on 7th Avenue and headed back toward 23rd and 10th.

'So what was that all about?' I asked.

'I wanted to see if a certain car was parked on that block.'

Certain car? I wondered if she'd been checking up on her pimp or on one of the other girls in his stable. But again I was wrong.

'What's so special about that car?'

'There's one car the cops use to pick up the girls,' she replied. 'If it's parked there that means they're done for the night.'

There's a police precinct on that block and nearly all the parking spaces there are reserved for their own vehicles. Finally I understood what had been going on.

'So was it there?'

'Yeah, it was,' she said with a sly smile.

'And this means you and the rest of the girls can work out there for the rest of the night and not have to worry about getting busted?'

'You got it, Mister Taxi Driver!'

Little had I suspected when this streetwalker entered my cab that I was dealing with a member of the elite Hooker Reconnaissance Unit, an urban guerilla squad which is trained to penetrate behind enemy lines to obtain the vital intelligence necessary to the survival of her company. Yes, they're a tough bunch of broads. And I hear they even have a motto: 'Tits, Ass – *and Guts*!'

Dying to get there

There are two things that hardly ever happen in taxicabs: birth and death. We do hear of stories in the news every once in a while of women who give birth in cabs, it is true. But this is extremely rare because the female body normally takes many hours to deliver a baby and there's plenty of time to get to the hospital.

But it's a bit more surprising that more people don't drop dead in cabs. Although sudden birth may not happen, sudden death does. Yet I've never heard of someone actually dying in a cab. In fact, it was a possibility that never even crossed my mind until a certain Type Three showed up on a Sunday evening in April, 1996 in lower Manhattan's Financial District.

He was a sixty-something man whose scruffy beard, unkempt gray hair and well-worn baseball cap gave him a rather haggard appearance. He asked me if I would take him to a hotel near Rutherford, New Jersey – a great ride for a taxi driver since it's an out-of-town job and, as such, it's done off the meter. The price of the ride is whatever we agree on and the deal we quickly struck was for $60 including tolls. That was good money and I was a happy cabbie.

I made a couple of turns and was heading for the Holland Tunnel when I noticed in the mirror that something was very wrong with this guy. His body was moving violently from left to right and his face was grimacing, apparently in great pain. It could not be ignored.

'Sir,' I asked, 'are you all right?'

'I just had a heart attack,' he blurted out in a tone of disgust.

It was one of those moments when you can't really believe what you just heard even though you know you just heard it. The shock wave kind of paralyzes you for a moment.

'You just had a *heart attack*?' I repeated. 'Shouldn't I take you to a hospital?'

His response was one of the great comeback lines of all time: '*I'm comin' from the hospital*,' he said. 'Those motherfuckers don't know what they're doing. I'd rather die in my hotel room.'

In fact, I had picked him up just a block away from the Beekman Downtown Hospital. My immediate response, which I think would be anybody's immediate response, was to try to get him to change his mind.

'Well, how about if I take you to a different hospital?' I asked.

'Just drive me to my fucking hotel!' he snarled back. Clearly the man had already considered this option and had decided to reject it. He was going to his hotel room and that was that. I drove on.

Now of all the types of uncomfortable rides that theoretically could be taken in a taxicab, here was a new category: the passenger who may drop dead at any minute. I looked at him again in the mirror as we moved along. He was in agony, continuing to move from side to side and clutching his chest. Then the pain would seem to subside and he would sit there relatively calmly for a bit.

I considered driving him to a hospital against his will, but I knew that if I did that, as soon as we came to a stop, he would get out, tell me to go fuck myself, and find himself another taxi. That was definitely the kind of guy he was. So it was either take him to New Jersey or lose him and lose the sixty bucks.

I decided to take him.

We entered the Holland Tunnel, the point of no return. Before we were halfway through, his writhing returned and was accompanied by moans of pain. I was becoming increasingly concerned that he was not going to make it and started to consider what I would do if he keeled over on the seat. I didn't know cardiac resuscitation and this was before the age of cell phones, so the only thing I could think of was to find a hospital. But then another thought occurred to me.

Wait a minute, if this guy dies, what about my fare? Do I charge for the whole ride to Rutherford or just from the point where he expired? And do I have the right to take my payment from his wallet? What about my tip? Should I give myself a normal, fifteen to twenty percent? Or should I be compensated for the trauma to my own psyche and throw myself a fifty? And if I do decide to take my money out of his wallet, should I do it before I get him to a hospital or after we get there? Hmmmm… I looked at the guy again in the mirror and this time I noticed that his baseball cap was kind of cool. The thought of keeping it crossed my mind but I quickly reprimanded myself for having even thought such a thing. But, hell, didn't I deserve it?

We drove on.

I considered trying to start a conversation with him, thinking that maybe if I could keep him talking he wouldn't die. People don't die in the middle of a sentence, right?

'So what brings you to New York?' I asked.

'What?'

'You're from out of town, right?'

'Man, just get me to my hotel, okay?'

So much for that. I couldn't think of anything else to say or do and resigned myself to the possibility of his imminent demise. Nevertheless, I drove well above my normal speed, trying to reduce the odds of his dying in the cab by reducing the time that he would be in it. The thought occurred to me of how perfectly ironic it would be if I lost control of the taxi and he wound up dying in a car wreck. Or, better yet, if I had a heart attack myself from the stress of worrying about the guy and *I* died, but *he* lived. But none of that happened. I got him to his hotel in another fifteen minutes, still breathing.

As I pulled into the driveway I thought I'd make one last attempt to convince him to seek medical treatment. I brought the cab to a stop and turned around to speak, but he was already out the door. He came over to my side of the cab, handed me seventy dollars without so much as breaking stride, and disappeared into the lobby.

Like the 'just drive' woman whose story I never learned, I wonder to this day if the guy survived through the night or died right there in his hotel room. And, if he did die, what about the maid who discovered his body in the morning? Did she take *her* tip from his wallet?

And what about that baseball cap?

While she sleeps

Of course, not all rides with Type Threes are trouble. Sometimes, in fact, extreme behavior can come up aces for a taxi driver. It happened one night in August, 1994, at around half past nine when a thirty-something man hailed me in lower Manhattan and asked if I would take him to Fort Lee, New Jersey. After a quick round of bargaining we agreed on $40 for the trip and we were on our way. Now, if that is a great ride, and it is, let me tell you what is an extraordinarily superb ride: about two minutes into the trip, he leaned forward in the back seat and with a voice slightly louder than a whisper (just to be sure he couldn't be overheard) he said…

'You want to go to Atlantic City?'

Cha-ching!

The timing was perfect. It's a four to five hour trip to Atlantic City and back, so if someone wanted to do this ride at, say, one in the morning, I wouldn't be able to get the cab back to the garage on time. But nine-thirty was fine. I drove to the Holland Tunnel and we were on our way to his new destination. But some tricky negotiation still needed to be done. We agreed on two hundred for the ride – that was the easy part – but then he said he wanted me to wait for him and drive him back to his place in Fort Lee when he was finished gambling.

'You're not going to stay in a hotel?' I asked.

'No,' he replied, *'I've got to get back before my wife wakes up.'*

Oh.

We had a little dilemma. On a ride like this, I've got to be paid in advance. You can't take the chance that your passenger will give you the slip once you arrive in Timbuktu. The problem from his perspective was how would he know that, once paid, I would not just take off? The truth is I wouldn't have done that, but how could he know? He felt I needed an incentive to be sure I'd be there to get him back to Fort Lee before, uh, his wife woke up. After a little thought he came up with a brilliant solution. He would pay me the two hundred up front and in addition to that he would cut me in for ten percent of his winnings, should he win.

I accepted his offer but only on the condition that we would have to leave the casino at one-thirty sharp. Any later than that and I'd be late getting back to the garage. He agreed and two hours later, at eleven-thirty, we arrived at the parking lot at Resorts and walked into the casino together. He sat himself down at a $25 blackjack table and asked me to check in with him every half hour. That was no problem, I said, and I took off into the casino to consider what I ought to do with the two hundred dollars that had recently arrived in my pocket.

I'm no kind of gambler – I work too hard for my money – so I decided to just stroll around and throw an occasional quarter into the slot machines, giving myself a $40 loss limit. Glancing over at him every once in a while from a distance, I couldn't get over the idea that, hey, that guy sitting over there at that $25 blackjack table? He's working for me! It was a no-lose situation in a casino where a whole science has been developed to basically guarantee that you will, in fact, lose. How great was that? Cha-ching!

My own gambling proceeded as it normally does on one of my rare visits to a casino – I was doing just a bit worse than breaking even. An hour in, I was about $10 in the red at a particular slot machine that caught my fancy – Hugh Hefner surrounded by a couple of Playboy bunnies urging me to keep the party going. When I reluctantly broke away from their hospitality for my second check-in, I found my guy was doing quite well in his own part of town. All smiles, he handed me four $25 chips as a reward-in-advance for my sticking with him. Who needed Hugh Hefner? Cha-ching-a-ding-ding!

At one-thirty, by then down $25 at slots but up $300 in passengers, I arrived at his table to collect him. Not needing any nudging, he immediately gathered his chips and walked off to cash out. While he was getting his money I had a little chat with the pit boss, who was amused that somebody would hail a cab on the street in Manhattan and suddenly take off for Atlantic City. I asked how he'd done at blackjack and was impressed that the pit boss knew the answer – he was up $700. So again I was a winner. I'd done better than the ten percent that had originally been offered me.

At 4 a.m., after a cheerful ride back, we arrived at his house on a quiet street in Fort Lee. As we said goodbye, I told him that I hoped his wife was a heavy sleeper.

'That's why I married her,' he said.

'I'll get out here'

Whether a passenger is a Type Three or just a normal person trying to get from Point A to Point B, there is one short sentence a cab driver doesn't want to hear when he's sitting in a hopeless, unmoving traffic jam:

'I'll get out here.'

It means that the driver is about to be sitting there by himself and will cease to make at least a little bit of money from the waiting time that's a part of the operation of the meter. Of course, it doesn't help matters in this situation if the person sitting in the back seat – who appeared to be just a regular human being when he got in the cab – turns out to be a raving lunatic.

He was a skinny guy with a pale complexion, dark hair, and was wearing what appeared to me to be a cheap suit. He jumped in on a Wednesday evening around 5 p.m. in Midtown, back in 1980. I know it's not kind to say it, but if I had to make a snap judgment about this person, I probably would have said 'loser'. He just had an air of anxiety about him. But there are a million guys like that. Just because he looks like he's a bit stressed out doesn't mean you expect him to explode.

'Please, please, driver,' he whined pathetically the moment the door closed, 'please, can you take me to Astoria in Queens?'

I hadn't said a word and already he was begging me.

Now, a fare out of Manhattan in the evening rush hour is horrible. You have to leave Manhattan (an island) at a snail's pace *with* a passenger – that's bad enough – but then you have to return to Manhattan at a snail's pace *without* a passenger, and that's complete misery because it's money lost. Nevertheless, I found myself feeling sorry for him. Sure, the rules say I have to take a passenger anywhere he wants to go, but it's easy enough to make up some excuse if you really don't want the fare – 'Sorry, buddy, my temperature light keeps coming on. I'm gonna have to bring this wreck back to the garage or it's gonna overheat.' Or some such.

But I thought if I refused this guy it might be the last straw for him and he'd probably throw himself in front of a truck or something. Actually I would be saving his life here.

I stepped on the gas and we were on our way.

The best route to Astoria from Manhattan is the 59th Street Bridge, which has both an upper and a lower level. To help accommodate the flow of traffic out of the city during the evening rush hours, the bridge in those days used to have both sides of the upper level going in the outbound direction from Manhattan. (Normally, of course, one side goes in and one side goes out.) I headed to the nearest entrance to the upper level at 62nd Street and in a flash we were on the ramp leading onto the bridge.

Immediately the traffic came to a complete stop. It was worse than usual, really bad. After a minute or two of barely moving an inch, I thought I'd pass some time by making conversation with my passenger. I glanced in the mirror and started to talk sports, but I quickly realized that I didn't have a conversationalist on my hands here, I had a nut.

He had his arms spread wide open and was pressing them against the rear seat as if he were holding it in place. His eyes were darting back and forth like a cuckoo clock. Dumbfounded, I stared at him through the mirror for a few moments, and then he spoke:

'Can't… you… drive… faster?' he gasped. And then in a pathetic, squeaky whine: *'Please… please… please?'*

I knew instinctively that he was so freaked out that he couldn't be reasoned with and that the only way to handle him would be to patronize him as if he were a child.

'It's okay, pal,' I said, 'it'll start moving soon. Calm down, it's all right. It's just the stupid evening rush hour traffic.'

His arms remained glued to the seat.

'I'm… claustrophobic… oh, please…'

'Don't worry, buddy. We'll be okay. Try to relax.'

'… *please…*'

Talking to the guy was useless. He was inconsolable, even though there was nothing to be inconsolable about. We crawled along for a couple more excruciatingly long minutes, barely putting a dent in our journey across the endless bridge. He continued to move around in the back but I could no longer bring myself to even look at him. I decided to quit this job and become a ditch digger, an alligator wrestler, a dentist – anything but this. And then I heard the dreaded words:

'I'll get out here.'

I turned and glared at him in disbelief.

'What do you mean?' I asked.

'I… I want to get out right here… please.'

'What are you going to do, *walk*? We're in the middle of the bridge!!!'

'The other side… it's moving faster.'

I looked over at the other side of the bridge which, along with our side, was also headed outbound. Indeed, the traffic was going faster over there. Maybe one mile per hour faster, but it was faster.

The meter was at $3. He handed me three bills, opened his door and got out of the cab. He then climbed over the railing that divides the two sides of the bridge and, to my astonishment, *immediately found an available cab*, which stopped for him. He got into it and, as soon as he did so, the traffic on that side of the bridge, as if on cue, began to move along at a decent pace. In a few moments both he and his new cab were gone from sight.

It took me another fifteen minutes to get across the damned bridge and another fifteen minutes to turn around and come back to Manhattan across the damned bridge again. Without doubt I had been singled out by the God of Vengeance to answer for sins I must have committed but now knew not what they may have been nor if they warranted anything like the merciless retribution I had been subjected to. What kind of a raw deal is that?

But maybe I shouldn't complain. At least I got paid.

Which is not always the case…

6

Fare Beaters

In New York we pick people up right off the street. There's no way of knowing who they are or whether or not they intend to pay the fare. We just take them where they want to go and hope at the end of the ride that cash will be tendered for the service that was rendered.

But it doesn't always work out that way, does it?

That's why a cabbie must always have his radar out for Mister C.U. Later and his female companion, Miss Sumotha Time. Most passengers pass through the filter without even making a blip on the screen. Two middle-aged businessmen going to a restaurant? Nothing to worry about. A little old lady returning home from the Metropolitan Opera (or a *big* old lady, come to think of it)? Don't even give it a second thought. Actually, the potential fare beaters fall into four categories: a) kids, b) drunks, c) the insane and d) born criminals.

Let's take them in order. When I say 'kids' I mean teenagers. There's no such thing as a child under the age of twelve riding alone or only with other children of the same age in a taxi. Never happens. But between the ages of about thirteen to nineteen, from a taxi driver's perspective – unless it's a rich kid from the American Aristocracy (Park Avenue or 5th Avenue) – you're in a danger zone. It's beyond their normal means for a middle class or inner city teenager to be traveling via taxicab. So immediately the suspicion is that the fare isn't a problem for them because they're not planning on paying it. One's antennas come out.

'Drunks' may be so out of it that they don't realize that they have no money on them. They get to the end of the ride and then discover to their own amazement that all they have in their pocket is a one dollar bill. Or possibly the money is somewhere on their person but the condition they're in makes finding it improbable. (Unless a cop appears on the scene. It's amazing how a completely plastered person is able to sober up enough to find his cash when the police arrive.) Anyway, it's not usually an intentional rip-off, but the result is the same.

'Insane' is a matter of degree. Nearly everyone is somewhat screwed up, but in this context I'm thinking of passengers who are institutional bait, not merely a member of the wide variety of eccentrics who populate the island. The guy gets in the cab, he seems all right and tells you where he wants to go, but halfway to his destination he suddenly says,

'I'm being followed by circus clowns. I just want you to know that I'm being followed by circus clowns.'

Oh, and by the way, he has no money – although with a fruit like this the money issue seems to fade into insignificance rather quickly.

And then there are the 'born criminals'. Here is the lowest form of human life next to a Red Sox fan, the person who has no excuse for ripping off a cab driver except that he's a mean-spirited, all-his-life-out-exchange, conniving, greed-head piece of feces. Really, what kind of deep-down, bedrock hostility must a person possess in order to plan out his little crime and then commit that crime on someone who has just given him personal service? It's not like he's shoplifting in a department store. That would be relatively impersonal. This is *personal.* Kids, drunks and the insane can be tolerated to some degree, but being taken for a sucker by *this guy* really stings.

The coat

In New York in 1977, the year I started driving a cab, it didn't take long to encounter a rip-off artist. The city was a wilder place in those days, but also quite possibly the potential fare beater is tipped off by a new cabbie's lack of street smarts, which I believe criminals are very well aware of. Any long-time taxi driver will tell you that the number of times he was beaten for a fare was much greater when he was still new at it.

That was certainly the case with me. The very first time I can remember being taken for a sucker was a ride I took from Queens, through a toll at the Midtown Tunnel (which *I* paid), and then eventually downtown to the East Village. My fare was a talkative male in his twenties who, when he got in the cab, was wearing a brown and white fur coat, unusual apparel for a guy. We were discussing the upcoming baseball season while driving down 2nd Avenue in Manhattan when he asked if we could stop at a deli. I said 'sure' and out he went without paying what was already on the meter. I wasn't concerned that he wouldn't return, however, because he left his coat on the back seat.

He soon returned to the cab with a brown paper bag in hand, which presumably held the sandwich he'd said he wanted. We continued down the avenue to the East Village and made a left onto St Mark's Place. Suddenly my passenger saw a smoke shop and apologetically asked me to pull over again so he could buy a pack of cigarettes. Since he'd already built up some rapport between us and had demonstrated his trustworthiness by leaving his coat in the cab, I didn't think twice about agreeing to this second favor.

It took me about a minute to start to become suspicious. I realized that when he left the cab he had walked *behind* the point where we'd stopped and that, not only was he out of sight, but I also hadn't bothered to notice what, if any, shop he'd entered. And then I discovered a particularly disturbing clue on the back seat.

The coat was not there.

I hoped that the reason he'd taken it was because he'd found it a bit too chilly the first time he'd left the cab. But even that thought was a sign of my own inexperience. After ten minutes of waiting I had to come to grips with the fact that I'd been made a fool of and it had cost me not only the time I'd lost but also the gasoline I'd used and the toll which I had paid.

I considered the trouble this guy had gone to in order to beat the fare. He'd been conversational. He had set me up with the coat. He deliberately had me stop on a one-way, crowded street and had walked away in the direction opposite to the flow of traffic, making it impossible for me to back up in order to keep him in sight.

It was a slap in the face. But it was also a learning experience. I vowed to use the knowledge I'd gained to not be victimized again.

Not long after this incident a young lady, also quite chatty, asked me to stop at a deli in mid-ride so she could run in and get a pack of cigarettes. This time I was careful to pull up right next to the store so I could keep an eye on the door. Five minutes went by. I started to become concerned, but not too concerned because, hell, where could she go? After another five minutes of waiting I nevertheless suspected that something was wrong. It never takes a full ten minutes to get something from a deli while a cab is sitting outside with the meter running. So I walked into the place to see what was taking so long.

To my amazement, the young lady was nowhere to be found. What *was* to be found, however, was a second door on the opposite side of the deli that led out onto the adjoining street.

Ouch!

But it was another lesson learned. Eventually I realized that I needed to have a firm policy in place to handle these types of fare beaters. And that policy is simply this: I say to the passenger who says he wants to leave and then (presumably) come back,

'No offense, but if you're going to leave the cab I need to have what's on the meter before you go. Over the years I've been ripped off by some of the most respectable-looking people you can imagine, so please don't take it personally.'

That usually handles any potential problems. But some of these people know how to find and exploit your weaknesses. Like the particularly attractive and somewhat drunk blonde who announced at the end of a ten-dollar ride to the Upper East Side that she didn't have any money and asked if it would be okay if she went up into her very high-rise, luxury apartment building to get the fare.

'I'll be back in five minutes,' she said, '*pinky promise.*'

And with that she presented her little finger to me through the partition window in order to invite my own little finger to join it in a sacred bond, which my little finger did.

After ten minutes of waiting I began to feel the sting of being had, but there was hope. The building had a doorman and he surely would know which apartment she lived in. So into the lobby I went, only to be told by this doorman that he had no idea who she was exactly, only that she'd been in and out of the place a few times and he assumed she was staying in a friend's apartment. And he didn't know which apartment that was.

So much for the sanctity of the pinky promise.

As years went by, however, it became more and more difficult to fool me. Not only had I become wise to the tricks, but in the mid-'90s the Taxi and Limousine Commission created one of its rare smart rules. A regulation was enacted requiring all New York taxis to be equipped with two secret 'help' signals – a circular, flat, orange light in the rear and another one behind the grille in the front. When the driver flips a silent switch this light starts flashing and becomes a call for help to the police.

One night a woman was giving me the runaround about needing to find her 'cousin' somewhere on 10th Avenue before she could pay the fare. It was a ruse and I knew it. So I flicked on the 'help' switch and, sure enough, before a minute had gone by a police cruiser pulled up behind us. I stopped the cab in the middle of the street and two cops emerged from their car and walked slowly toward us, one of them with his gun drawn. Amazingly, the woman who had no cash soon found that she had the money for the ride.

So it turns out you have to be either very bold and or very original to pull a fast one on a veteran cabbie. And it doesn't hurt if you're both…

The slip

At 2 a.m. one night in May, 2003 I picked up a twenty-something, kind of tough-looking guy in Times Square and began driving him toward his destination in Harlem, to 118th Street between 7th and 8th Avenues. When I get a fare to a part of town that is on the rough side (although Harlem by that time was in mid-gentrification) at a time of day when there aren't too many people around, and my passenger strikes me as potentially threatening, I make it a firm policy to start a conversation with that passenger. I will talk about anything, and I will keep talking to him until I reach a decision about him. The reason I do this is to feel him out, to get a read on what his intentions may be. In cold fact, I am trying to determine if he plans on holding me up. If I still feel uncomfortable after talking to him or trying to talk to him, I will find a way to get rid of him before we get to his destination. It's a policy that may have saved my life once or twice. And I've never been held up.

So I started being chatty with this particular guy and found that he was a punk but, as is almost always the case, that he was relatively okay. By 'relatively' I mean that I felt certain after communicating with him that he wasn't going to pull a gun on me.

Of course, that doesn't mean he intended to pay for the ride.

When we arrived at 118th Street the meter was at $10.60, not a tremendous amount of money but enough to make me care if I didn't receive it. He directed me to a brownstone in the middle of the block which had two or three people sitting around on the building's stoop. Then he committed a passenger's no-no.

'I've gotta get the money from one of those guys up there,' he said. 'I'll be back in a second.'

Now, if this had been 1977 I would have said, 'Sure, no problem.' But by 2003 I was many years removed from making that mistake. If passengers are being straight with you, they do not announce at the end of the ride that they don't have the money to pay the fare. They announce it at the beginning of the ride. So my reaction was immediate and it was unflinching.

'Negative,' I said. And with that one word I slammed the partition shut and locked it. Then, before he could open the door and run off, I started moving the cab forward.

'Let's find a cop,' I said.

The strategy here is to prevent the passenger from opening the door and running away by keeping the taxi moving – even running red lights – until a police car can be found or a police precinct reached. With the partition closed the cab becomes a moving cage and it is quite startling to a passenger to suddenly find himself in this predicament.

'Hey, man,' he pleaded, 'you gonna get me arrested for ten bucks?'

'It's not the ten bucks,' I called back to him, 'it's not letting you make an ass out of me.' Which was completely the truth of the matter. It's not the money. It's the principle.

I made a right turn on 7th Avenue and started looking for the police. Driving at about fifteen miles per hour – just enough speed to prevent him from leaping out – my eyes scanned the area two blocks ahead, left to right, right to left, hoping to find the elusive cop. But, as the saying goes, you can't find a cop when you need one, and so when we arrived at Central Park North, where 7th Avenue ends, I was still cop-less.

I turned right and headed back toward 8th Avenue. I started thinking about where the nearest precinct might be, but my passenger surprised me by announcing that he had the cash after all.

'It was in my coat pocket, man, I forgot that I had anything in there,' he said. 'Here, here…'

And with that he pulled open the small Plexiglas slot that's used to make money exchanges between passenger and driver when the partition is closed, and he placed his payment in it.

I was surprised but not completely shocked. Criminal-type passengers quite often have a way of producing payment when the heat is turned on and they know they've lost the game.

I felt an immediate sense of satisfaction in having spotted the guy for what he was and successfully preventing him from making me his latest cab driver sucker.

I slowed the cab down to about ten miles per hour and turned my body around to get the money from the slot while keeping my head straight and my eyes on the road. As I did this, two things happened at the same time:

1. The guy opened his door, jumped out of the cab *while it was still moving*, and started running back toward 7th Avenue in the opposite direction from which the cab was headed, and

2. I discovered that his 'payment' consisted of a folded-up piece of cardboard.

I started to swing the cab around into a U-turn, but was delayed by an oncoming vehicle. Then I found there wasn't enough room to make a U-turn, so it became a three-point turn. When I finally was able to complete the maneuver I peered through the windshield to try to see him, but by this time he'd disappeared into the shadows of Harlem, never to be seen again.

This serves to illustrate the fact that the best way to beat a fare, and I write this on the assumption that people who would beat a fare would not be buying a book written by a taxi driver (although they might steal it), is simply to run in the opposite direction as fast as you can, preferably on a narrow, one-way street. A cabbie cannot stop his taxi in the middle of the road, turn off the engine, roll up the windows, lock the doors, and then hope to catch you in a footrace.

But it wouldn't be a bad idea for a driver to have his track shoes on, anyway…

'Don't mess with the Bronx'

The night of the week when you're most likely to encounter the teenage fare beater is Saturday. This is because Saturday is date night and a fourteen- or fifteen-year-old could conceivably be out on a big date and splurging on taxicab transportation. So when a teenager hails you on a Saturday you're alert for the rip-off, but you're thinking at the same time that it's probably okay.

Which is what I thought in the summer of 2006 when three kids, two guys and a girl, got in my cab at 108th Street and Amsterdam Avenue, the area where the Upper West Side melds into Harlem. These kids were African-Americans and I could tell by their immediate destination (further uptown), their dress and their language with each other that they were from the inner city, not a middle-class neighborhood. This is a further red flag to a taxi driver as the economics alone make riding in a cab an extravagance for them. So I was uneasy with it from the start.

As it turned out, the two guys got out at 122nd Street and 1st Avenue and the girl wanted to continue on up to the Bronx. This was yet another red flag to me, as it meant the cost of the ride was going from medium-priced to high-priced. The girl was about fifteen and kids from the inner city, traveling alone and therefore not splitting the fare with other passengers, just do not spend money that way.

She told me her destination was an obscure street near Castle Hill Avenue, a road with which I was familiar. And then came another warning sign: she told me that the way that she wanted to go was a route that was totally out of the way. It would have added about $10 to the ride unnecessarily. When I replied that I knew a shorter, faster and cheaper way to go, she said 'okay' but didn't really seem to care.

I noted the outpoint. Why would a fifteen-year-old inner city kid *not* be concerned about what route the taxi driver took? Uh, could it be that she had no plans of paying for the ride?

My tension was growing. This ride was all wrong. I considered the option of just blatantly telling her I had a feeling I wasn't going to get paid and demanding that she show me her money. But the repercussions of doing this would be unpleasant. There were already about $13 on the meter and she could tell me to go fuck myself and get out without paying. Or maybe she *did* have the money which would make the remainder of the ride uncomfortable to say the least. So I decided to do what I always do when I am ill at ease with a passenger.

I communicate.

I started chatting it up and to my surprise I found her to be conversational and friendly. We spoke easily about various mundane topics like television shows and movies and before long she had won me over in a trust sense and I was glad I hadn't insulted her by doubting her intention to pay for the ride. I didn't even become overly suspicious when at one point she excused herself from our conversation to get on her cell phone. She spoke with her mother and told her in a voice just loud enough for me to hear that she was about three minutes away and that she'd come to the window to get the money.

She'd come to the window to get the money? Well, I didn't like the idea of that, but it was something that did happen every once in a while. It brought to mind a time when a passenger had received her cab fare in a little purse that had been dropped down to the sidewalk from the seventh floor of an apartment building, kind of an urban airmail. So this kind of money relay, although unusual, was not completely unheard of.

Still, I didn't like it.

As we got closer to her destination, she continued to charm me.

'Watch out for the bump,' she warned as we approached a particularly insidious protrusion in the street. It's nice when a passenger who knows the terrain is looking out for you. This was a section of the Bronx that is, like many inner city areas of New York, a place where the roads always seem to be in need of repair.

I slowed down to avoid the bump and then was directed into a narrow parking lot that led up to a large apartment building. But it wasn't just any apartment building – it was a project building. The 'projects' are low-rent, government-subsidized housing areas that are as ghetto as ghetto gets. The realization that she was bringing me there suddenly raised my taxi driver alert level to bright red. This was an unwelcome development in the story line.

What happened next was this:

a) the fare showing on the meter was just over $20,

b) she told me she had to go to a window on the ground floor of the building that was about a hundred feet away from us in order to get the money from her mother,

c) since I had been prepared for this I said 'okay',

d) she got out of the cab and walked toward the building,

e) while watching her carefully I instinctively rolled up the windows,

f) instead of walking to one of the first-floor windows, she walked toward a passageway that led into a dark area,

g) I immediately turned off the engine, opened the door, locked the locks, stepped out of the cab, put the key in my pocket, and slammed the door shut,

h) she began running into the dark area,

i) knowing that the cab was secured, I took off after her at full speed, angered by the realization that the 'conversation' with her 'mother' was a set-up, as was her pretended concern for my well-being.

So the chase was on. The dark area turned out to be a hallway that led into a courtyard which was surrounded by two other project buildings. The aroma of marijuana permeated the air in there, and I realized I was entering an inner-city sanctum and *a white, middle-aged man's no-man's-land.* But that didn't stop me from continuing forward in my quest for justice. The game was afoot (literally), as Holmes would have said to Watson.

What came next was a scene right out of a cop show. In fact, even as it was happening I had the feeling I was in a movie. I looked all around at this unexpected environment searching for the fugitive, but she had disappeared. Then I heard the sound of a door closing with a loud 'thud'. I knew from that sound that she'd entered the project building on my right.

I ran to the entrance of the building, opened the door, and found myself in an empty hallway. But far down on the right I could hear the sound of running footsteps, then the sound of another door opening and slamming closed. I ran down the hallway in the direction of the sound, then found myself in an adjoining hallway with a door at the end of it. I ran to that door, opened it, and discovered that I was back in the courtyard again. And there she was, halfway across the courtyard, running with the long strides of an Olympic sprinter in the two hundred meter dash.

I gave chase, but realized in just a few steps that this was a race I was not going to win – she was just much too fast for me. She exited the courtyard on the opposite side from where we'd entered and ran out onto the street and out of sight. By the time I got to the other side of the courtyard, all I could see was a street scene without a fare beater on it. She was gone and the game was lost.

I turned around and started walking back through the courtyard in the direction of my taxi, but before I'd taken ten steps in that direction I realized I had a new game to play – making it back to my cab unscathed. My chase scene had been witnessed by residents who'd been hanging out in the courtyard, and their eyes were upon me.

I understood immediately that I was in a danger zone. What had these people just seen? A middle-aged white man chasing a young black girl in their own space. I don't know all the rules of the ghetto culture but I did know instinctively that I'd just broken one of them.

A young, particularly tough-looking thug-type came forward and stood in my way, having elected himself the president of the Community Board of Inquiry. A few others stood behind him. The distance between where I was standing and my cab was suddenly ten miles. Without any words being spoken, I knew I was expected to make a statement.

'I'm a cab driver,' I said. 'She just beat me for a $20 fare.'

The jury listened to my explanation and through the osmosis of nods and gestures returned their verdict: I would be granted safe passage out of the courtyard. But the fellow in charge had something to say before I began the long walk back to my cab.

'*Don't mess with the Bronx*,' he said.

Arrested development

The Bronx. I must admit that even after all these years, I still don't know that borough very well. And when a passenger gets in the cab and announces the Bronx as his destination, inside I cringe. For one thing, it's almost always a 'money lost' ride. You never get a fare back to Manhattan from the Bronx. And the other thing, since most of the borough is inner city, is the cultural friction that often exists between the taxi driver and the 'hood'. My 'off-duty' light goes on when I arrive there, my doors are locked, and my radar is always on the alert for some kind of unwelcome occurrence.

Like the night of May 20, 2004. During the course of an otherwise ordinary shift, a normal-looking, middle-aged gentleman entered my cab at 69th Street and Lexington Avenue in Manhattan at 11 p.m. He was well dressed and rather conservative in appearance and it occurred to me that he might be coming from Hunter College, which is right there on Lex.

He said in a soft voice that he wanted to go to a certain street in the Bronx, a street I didn't know. So I told him I would need directions, to which he replied that it would be okay, he could show me the way. The first thing was to get on the FDR Drive and take the Willis Avenue Bridge. That was no problem, so off we went.

I paid no special attention to this passenger as we began the ride. He was not the conversational type and his appearance and demeanor posed no threat or indication that this was anything but a mundane trip to a part of the city where I'd rather not be. I would simply need his help to get him to his specific destination, then I would have a little empty-time before getting back to Manhattan.

It took just over ten minutes to get to the Willis Avenue Bridge, which lets you out in the South Bronx. We drove for a few minutes on Willis Avenue, then began making a left here and a right there onto streets I had no familiarity with. After a few minutes of this I had lost my sense of direction and knew only that I was somewhere in the South Bronx and that getting back to the highway was going to take up more of my time than I had expected. I continued to follow my passenger's directions until we arrived at a certain bleak-looking road and he asked me to stop. I pulled over and waited for payment to arrive from the back seat, but instead what arrived was this statement:

'I have no money to pay you.'

'What?'

'I have no money.'

I was incredulous. Fare beaters always have an excuse or suddenly need to leave the cab to 'get the money' or *something.* Normal-looking, middle-aged men don't just sit there and quietly announce that they have no money. I was angered but I was also curious.

'You mean you had me drive you all the way up here knowing that you had no money to pay the fare?' I asked sharply.

'That's right.'

This guy was amazing. There he sat in the back seat without

hostility, without fear, without defiance, simply stating flatly that he had used my services without any intention of paying for those services. This was indeed a first.

'Why?' I asked calmly.

'I want you to arrest me,' he said.

'*What?*'

'I want you to take me over there to the precinct and press charges against me,' he said as he pointed to the other side of the street. I looked where he'd indicated. In fact, there was a police precinct right there across the street.

I really couldn't believe this guy was for real.

'You want me to bring you to the precinct and press charges against you for, what, theft of services?'

'That's right.'

It's funny how one's own emotions can be altered by the significance attached to an action. Even though the actuality of the situation had not changed – meaning that the passenger was not going to pay for the ride – I no longer felt any sense of outrage because he wasn't trying to pull a fast one on me. In fact, what he was doing was the opposite of pulling a fast one. He wasn't trying to get something and then avoid the repercussions for not paying for it. He was *inviting* the repercussions. And this had the effect on me of nullifying my anger. I was no longer particularly concerned about the money I was losing. I just wanted to know what was up with this person.

'Why would I do that? I don't want to send you to jail,' I replied, beginning to feel some sympathy for him.

'You'd be doing me a favor,' he said.

'Why?'

'Because if I don't go to jail, someone is going to kill me,' he said without emotion. 'It's the only place where I can be safe.'

I looked at him in the mirror. The options passed quickly

through my mind: a) he was telling the truth, b) he was an actor practicing a scene on a real cab driver, or c) he was completely out of his freaking mind.

Of course, with a statement like that I wanted the whole story. So I delved. And what I learned was that he was under the firm belief that the boyfriend of his ex-wife was convinced that the world would be a better place if he were not in it and that if he returned to his home he would not live through the night. The boyfriend of his ex-wife was a jealous crazy-man, according to my passenger, and he had nowhere to run. Except jail. There he would be safe.

As bizarre as his story sounded, I could see that he was in a state of mind that wouldn't hear of there being any other solution. And for all I knew, every word he said was true and there wasn't any other solution, so who was I to try to talk him out of it? Still, my idea of helping somebody isn't to march him into a police station. I tried to tell him he could forget about the fare and, you know, good luck and goodbye. But he persisted, and finally he had me convinced. In what now seems like a scene from a comedy, I agreed to do him a favor by accompanying him into the precinct so he could be arrested. We exited the cab, I locked the doors, and we walked across the street toward the station house.

'Are you *sure* you want to do this?' I asked just before we reached the door. It was still hard for me to fathom that anyone would *want* to be arrested. He looked at me with utter resignation in his eyes.

'Thank you, man. I really appreciate this,' he replied.

We went in and approached an officer sitting behind a desk who looked like the person to speak to. As I began to talk I found myself somewhat at a loss for words. It was difficult for me to explain to him the reason for our entry into his castle.

'Uh, I'm a taxi driver and this gentleman got in my cab in

Manhattan and now says he has no money to pay the fare…'

'Okay.'

'He wants me to have him arrested.'

'Say what?'

'I don't want to have him arrested, but he talked me into bringing him in here.'

'Are you shitting with me?'

'Uh, no, I know this is weird. But he says he wants to be arrested.'

There was a long pause. I noticed we had been overheard by a couple of other cops in the vicinity and motion in the station house had been momentarily brought to a halt by the oddity of the circumstance. My passenger stepped forward and spoke.

'I have warrants,' he said.

It turned out these were the magic words. Suddenly the two or three cops in the background and the cop behind the desk came forward and put their hands on my passenger. They had him put his hands over his head and place them on the wall. They then patted him down and had him empty his pockets. Finding literally nothing on his person, including any money, they led him away to another part of the station house to be questioned.

I was stunned. Not being familiar with the jargon of the criminal justice system, I didn't immediately understand what the implications were of his statement to the police. I soon learned that 'having warrants' means you have *outstanding* warrants. In other words, it means the cops are already looking for you.

I was asked by one of the officers if I wanted to press charges. Of course, I said no. By this time I was completely sympathetic to the guy and would have gladly given him a free ride to wherever he may have wanted to go. But he had been taken away to be 'run through the system'.

The officer and I stepped outside onto the street and had a brief chat before I was on my way. I wanted to know what he thought would happen with him. He told me they would first establish his identity and see if, in fact, he did have any outstanding warrants. Depending on what they found he would either be held to face whatever charges he'd been previously arrested for, he'd be released, or, if they thought it appropriate, he'd be sent to a psychiatric facility, a possibility that I found disturbing as I would never want to think that I had any hand in sending anyone to one of those places.

'Do you suppose this whole thing could have been an elaborate way of beating a fare?' I asked the officer. 'I mean, do you think he could have gone into the precinct knowing that he *doesn't* have any outstanding warrants and also knowing that no cab driver is going to hang around filing a complaint? So it takes up some of his time but he winds up getting a free ride?'

The officer smiled at the thought.

'Well,' he said, 'that would be a long shot. But then again, you never know... this *is* New York City, after all.'

From Zurich, with love

Experiences like these can give a cab driver the opinion that the human race consists of cheats, two-faced sneaky bastards, outright lunatics and people who can run faster than you. My own outlook on the world wasn't helped by something that occurred on July 24, 1984.

I had just finished a late breakfast at a coffee shop in Greenwich Village and was getting into my cab to continue my shift when two young men approached me on the street. They asked a minute of my time so they could explain a peculiar situation they were in and offer me a deal. That sounded interesting so I lent them an ear. The one who did all the talking was a blond-haired fellow who said he was an American attending college in Zurich, Switzerland, and was in New York because his friend, a thin, dark-haired Moroccan, was an artist whose paintings were having a show at a gallery in Soho.

The story he told turned out to be more than a little intriguing. It went like this…

Just a little while earlier they had been walking down a nearby street in the Village when they were asked for help by an intoxicated man who was at a telephone booth and was holding a phone in his hand. In barely understandable drunk-talk he was able to communicate to them that he wanted one of them to get on the phone for him as he was too strung out to speak coherently with the party on the other end. The American kid obliged and found himself in conversation with a man who said he was a 'Doctor Rothman' who lived on Park Avenue near 75th Street.

Doctor Rothman told him that the drunk man on the street had three rare coins worth $2000 in his possession which belonged to him. Two days earlier, he said, his wife had been on her way to the bank with the coins where she'd intended to place them in their safe deposit box when she stopped at a restaurant to eat, placed her bag containing the coins on a chair, and found, when she'd finished her meal, that her bag was gone. The doctor was offering a $500 reward for their return, no questions asked. He didn't know if the drunk was the person who had stolen them or not, and he didn't care, but he did know that the guy was too incoherent to take directions to his apartment building. What he wanted them to do was to give the drunk some money for the coins and then come to his place on Park Avenue to collect the reward.

They agreed to the doctor's offer and were able to get the drunk to understand that they were willing to pay him for the coins so they could return them to their owner. The drunk wanted a hundred for them, but all they had on them was $56 which, after some haggling, the drunk accepted since apparently he felt this would be enough money to keep him boozed up for the rest of the day and maybe the next day, too.

So now they had the three coins in their possession, which they showed me. They were each displayed in their own little plastic window surrounded by a white, cardboard holder with writing on the cardboard describing the coin and its value. One of them was an Indian head penny and the other two were foreign coins which I didn't recognize.

The problem was that they'd given the drunk all their money and now had no means to get to the doctor's residence. And that's where I came in. The deal they offered me was that if I would drive them to the Park Avenue address, they would pay me what was on the meter plus a very generous tip after they'd gotten the reward money from the doctor. Would I do it?

Of course I would! I liked these guys and felt that participating in their adventure and seeing how it turned out would be well worth my time and effort, even if getting paid wasn't a certainty. So off we went toward the Upper East Side. I joked along the way that in the event that they didn't get the reward money, I would get to keep the Moroccan. I figured I could use him to paint my own apartment. They agreed.

It took us about fifteen minutes to get to Park Avenue and 75th Street. I stopped right in front of the building and the American, whose name I'd learned by this time was Scott, got out by himself and walked up to the entrance. He opened the door and spoke to the doorman there. And then a strange thing happened – the doorman started laughing! There was a little more conversation between them and then Scott turned around and walked back to the cab. I noticed that the doorman continued to have a huge grin on his face as he watched him depart.

It turned out my passengers had been the third and fourth suckers looking for 'Dr Rothman' that week. There was no such person. The drunk on the street had been an actor. The person on the telephone line had been an actor. The coins were of little value. They had been conned.

The three of us took it well. In fact, there were laughs all around. Things like this can quickly be looked at humorously as long, I suppose, as the losses aren't too great. They were out $56 and I was out the money for a fare (although technically I had gained a Moroccan, I reminded them), so it wasn't the end of the world. We were about to part ways when Scott, realizing he and his friend were about to be stranded on the Upper East Side, had a new idea and a new proposal for me. Would I be willing to extend myself a bit further by driving them down to their friend's apartment in the East Village? That's where they were staying and that's where their money was, which meant they could still pay me what they owed me.

How could I say no?

Twelve minutes later we arrived at the designated building on 6th Street between 1st and 2nd Avenues. But their friend wasn't home and his door was locked which meant that they couldn't get in and I wasn't going to get paid after all.

Well, it was easy enough to adopt a *c'est la vie* attitude about the whole thing. These guys were certainly not in the same category as the usual fare beater and I felt no sense of animosity or of being cheated by them. Scott asked me for my mailing address and promised to send me a check for the fare, a gesture which didn't really surprise me considering that the rapport had been created by our little adventure was quite high. We all shook hands and wished each other well. And off I drove to continue with my day.

I wondered if I would ever get that check. My instincts told me that I would, but the social façade that people use to get through life with other people can really fool you. How does a person behave when there is no possibility of repercussions for his actions? How much integrity do you really have when there's no one else around? That is the test of a human being.

I figured I should get the payment within two weeks if I was to get it at all. When a month went by and I still hadn't received it, I pretty much wrote it off mentally as a bad debt. In a monetary sense it was no big deal, of course, but it added one more shovelful of dirt onto the mountain of cynicism that accumulates over a lifetime. Make note: 'Even the nice ones cannot be trusted.'

Four months later, in the middle of December, I received a letter in the mail postmarked in Switzerland and addressed to 'The Trusting and Delightful Mr Eugene Salomon'. Inside the envelope was a check for the fare and a post card from Zurich which read:

> 'If I were a betting man, which I sometimes am, I would lay 100–1 that you had written off the fare of July 24th completely. There was this guy and his friend who had some cock and bull story of coins worth $2,000 and they wanted you to go to Park Avenue to collect the $500 reward. No reward and no money. You drove them back to their 'friend' in the Village to get paid and be on your way… but the fellow wasn't there. An exchange of shrugs, smiles, handshakes, and you drove away, resigned and accepting what the Fates would bring, saying there was a 50/50 chance…
>
> Sorry about the delay! I wish I were a millionaire who could reward your openness and kindness with a few thousand… but alas. Please receive my thanks, however, and best wishes. You were a kind and good soul amidst the sharks and piranhas of the city. Merry Christmas to you. Have a good 1985! Scott.'

Correction to 'make note': 'People are basically good. Always try to give them a chance to demonstrate their decency.'

7

Means of Exchange

Well, this whole painful subject of beating fares brings to mind the wider subject of exchange in general. I don't know if it ever really occurs to most people that all of civilization hinges on this one, basic principle: I do something for you and you do something for me. I bake you a pie and you mow my lawn. It's when I bake you a pie and you eat it without doing anything for me that the trouble begins.

In the taxi business you give someone a ride and they pay you with money. That's pretty simple, isn't it? To make it even simpler, taximeters have been invented which show you right there on the meter what the money exchange should be.

Or does it?

Well, I must admit that there's a flip side to the painful subject of fare beating and that's the painful subject of rigging the meter to make it run faster than it should. For example, there was a story in the papers here in New York years ago about a taxi driver who'd wired his cab so that whenever he pressed on his horn the meter clicked. That was a classic. And aside from funny meters, there's also the painful subject of 'taking the scenic route'. Particularly popular at the airports, this technique consists of going to Manhattan via Queens, Brooklyn *and* the Bronx.

But assuming there's no intention to deceive by either passenger or driver, what can be done when money is taken out of the equation? Let's say a passenger discovers as he arrives at his place of work in a taxicab that, to his horror, he has left his wallet at home and has no money to pay the fare. Or a passenger knows she has no money before getting into the taxi but has something else to offer in exchange. It can get quite creative.

A young woman, for example, once discovered at the end of a ride from Chelsea to the Lower East Side that she had only a dollar in her pocket, not nearly enough to pay what was on the meter. Leaving her friend in the cab with me as collateral, she went into her apartment building and soon returned with a tea kettle. It served me well for years. Another passenger had no money but he did have a bag full of books. That ride was paid for with two second-hand novels and a cookbook. Still another, en route to the Upper West Side from the Whole Foods store in Columbus Circle, realized she didn't have enough dough as we were halfway up Central Park West. Her solution: in addition to the money she did have, she paid me with a bag of cherries. Delicious!

Here's looking at you

There was one time when the idea of exchanging the ride for a service from the passenger was initiated by me. In conversation with a tourist who was going from Times Square to the West Village, it was mentioned that she was a dermatologist from Oregon. It so happened that at that time I had been wondering if a certain mole on my back could possibly be skin cancer and I had decided to have it checked out soon. So I struck a deal with my passenger: instead of paying me money for the ride I asked her to give me her professional opinion about the mole on my back. She cheerfully agreed (more delighted at the idea of such an exchange ever occurring than at the idea of saving a few dollars), so when we arrived at her destination I got out of the cab and took off my shirt, attracting the attention of several people and a couple of dogs passing by on Charles Street. My back was then thoroughly inspected and I was assured that the mole was not dangerous, making me quite happy not only that the news was good but also that a $9 taxi ride had been the exchange for a $90 doctor's visit. What a deal!

For a laugh

In the summer of 1990 I was hailed on 6th Avenue in Greenwich Village by an attractive young lady who was pregnant. Perhaps that's an understatement. Actually, she was *too* pregnant: her belly was so huge it looked like she would soon be giving birth to an elephant. I noticed, however, that she slid into the back seat with the grace of a gazelle. It raised an eyebrow.

'I want to go to Tompkins Square Park in the East Village,' she blurted out immediately, 'but, you know, I'm nine months pregnant and I don't have any money.'

This was so up front and fresh that I found it rather disarming. I pulled out from the curb and made a right on West 4th Street, not knowing how long I'd be willing to keep driving for no exchange, but at least for the moment showing her that I was willing to keep listening to her justifications for why it was okay not to pay.

'So what you're saying is that if you're pregnant you get everything for free?' I inquired.

She displayed a wry smile.

'Well, no,' she said, 'but I *can't* pay you and as you can see I'm nine months pregnant.'

Actually what I could see was that she was nine months *pillow*!

She was trying to use her gigantic bulge to push people's sympathy buttons and get stuff for free. Nevertheless, it was one of those times when you know someone is full of it, and the person knows that you know that she is full of it, but you don't care because of the entertainment value of the pretense. I continued driving.

'Well, you know, I have a strict policy when it comes to giving rides,' I said in a friendly way, 'and that is that everyone has to pay something. No free rides. Strict company policy.'

'Yeah, but I don't have any money, man.'

'Well, maybe you can think of something else to offer me in exchange for the ride,' I said. 'It doesn't *have* to be money.'

She thought about this for a few moments. Then, as we came to a red light at LaGuardia Place, she had an idea.

'How about a joke?' she asked.

A joke! I thought right away that it would be a fair enough exchange. For one thing, there was the novelty of it: perhaps in the history of taxi driving, no one had ever before paid for a ride with a joke. And for another thing, it was a short ride. If someone was going to Kennedy Airport from Manhattan and wanted to pay with a joke, the only joke would be the one on me. But this was just a shortie to the East Village. I decided to accept her offer.

'Well, okay,' I said, 'but it has to be a joke I haven't heard before. Wooden nickels and used jokes are not accepted in this taxi!'

She was up for the challenge.

'Okay,' she said. 'Here goes.' And with that, she told me her joke:

'Why was Six afraid of Seven?'

'Why?'

'Because Seven ate Nine.'

I had not heard that one before and it brought a smile. I told her I liked it and I thought that my daughter, who was seven at the time, would like it, too. And I told her that her fare had been paid.

In an interesting way this back and forth created a little bond between us. She saw that she had been able to give me something of value in order to receive something of value, and this at least for the moment had raised her self-esteem. She was no longer a cheat. She could contribute. And I was now a person who could be communicated with and could be trusted.

We began to talk and I learned enough of her story to understand how she came to be walking around Greenwich Village with a pillow under her dress. She was a middle-class kid who'd dropped out of some college that was somewhere else and had taken off with her artist boyfriend for New York City. They were both heavily into drugs and wound up establishing residence in Tompkins Square Park, which was something you could do in those days. I was able to get it across to her in a gentle way that she needed to make a decision to quit the shit, that the time for change had come for her, and that the only real change can come from within.

'I know,' she said, and she said it in a way that made me feel that she did indeed know it and that maybe she just needed the right person to tell her. Within a minute we arrived at the park and said our goodbyes.

'Thanks for the ride,' she said.

'Hey, thanks for the joke,' I replied.

She closed the back door, started to walk off, took a few steps, and then, before I could drive away, she turned around and said something else to me.

'I love you!' she called out with a big smile. I returned her smile, waved farewell, and headed off down Avenue A.

Looking back at it, she'd given me a joke which my daughter did indeed enjoy, a story which has been retold in my cab countless times, and a wonderful acknowledgment that I've never forgotten. Looks like *I* was the one who was short on the exchange factor here – she'd given me much more than I could ever have expected for a six-minute ride across town.

Having a cow

Cruising along Bleecker Street in Greenwich Village one chilly evening in November, 1989, a scruffy-looking guy, probably in his mid-thirties, came running up to my cab in a *big rush.* He jumped in the back seat and, as I started to accelerate, I noticed he had turned around and was looking out the rear window as if someone might be chasing after him.

'Make the light, man, make the light!' he cried out as we approached 7th Avenue South. I hate it when a passenger tries to tell me how to drive, so I just kept moving the cab at a pace I was comfortable with and we made the light anyway. The guy then turned around and faced forward.

'Take me to Little Italy,' he ordered. Ugh. I didn't like the tone of his voice. He hadn't made it through my 'friendly passenger' filter so I went into 'no conversation' mode and just drove downtown on the avenue in silence, knowing this was one of those rides that you just want to bring to a conclusion as quickly as possible. Only when I needed directions did I speak up.

'So where do you want to go down here?' I asked as we approached Little Italy on Grand Street.

He leaned forward in his seat and looked around through the windshield as if he was searching for a landmark.

'Make a left on Mulberry,' he commanded. I complied and stopped at a red light at the next intersection, Broome Street.

'Now what?' I asked.

'Make a left.'

I turned left when the light turned green and started to drive west on Broome at a slow clip.

'Now what?'

'Okay, stop here. I'll be right back.'

And with no further words spoken he opened his door and exited the taxi. This sets off a loud alarm in a cabbie's head. He'd left the cab too abruptly – something was up with this guy. I watched him carefully as he took a few steps on the sidewalk and noticed that he was carrying a shopping bag on one arm that seemed a bit heavy from the way he was holding it. He walked with his bag up to an Italian restaurant and entered the place. It was weird. Why would somebody walk into a restaurant with a shopping bag?

I waited for him to come out, which he did in about a minute. And then he committed a huge no-no. Instead of coming back to the taxi, he continued strolling down Broome Street and walked into a second Italian restaurant. It was a red alert. I left the taxi myself and waited on the sidewalk for him to come out, which he did in another minute.

'Okay, what's going on?' I asked confrontationally.

He looked at me with an expression of desperation and hopelessness.

'I don't have any money, man. I'm trying to sell these.'

And with that he opened his bag and showed me its contents. It was filled with packaged meats from the Gristedes supermarket. I realized immediately why he'd been in a big rush when he'd jumped in my cab: there was a Gristedes on that block and he'd just stolen the meats! I had been his getaway driver!

'You mean I have to wait for you to make a *sale* before I can get paid?' I asked with subdued anger. I should have been outraged but the situation was so absurd that I was finding it somewhat comical.

The guy knew he had a problem on his hands with me standing there, so he came up with an idea.

'Tell you what,' he said, 'why don't you take one of the meats as payment for the ride?'

I thought about it for a second and realized that under the circumstances it was a brilliant solution. The fare on the meter was $5.30, so I picked out a rib roast that had a $9.65 price tag on it, put it in the trunk for refrigeration, and then got back in the cab and drove off, leaving Mister Beef Brain and his bag of stolen meats standing there on Broome Street.

I guess there aren't too many good things that could be said about a thief, but there was one positive thing about this person that deserves to be noted – what with the difference between the price of the taxi ride and the price of the rib roast, it can't be denied that, regardless of his character flaws, the guy was an *excellent* tipper!

8

Hustlers, Hustlers, Hustlers

> Hustler: Informal. One who earns a living by energetic scheming, begging, or cheating.
> *(Macmillan Dictionary for Students)*

Perhaps New York City has always been a city of hustlers, but at the time when I started driving a cab in 1977 and going on through the early '90s, it seemed like there had been an invasion and the hustlers were approaching conquest. It may be an exaggeration, but perhaps not too much of one, to say that wherever you turned there seemed to be someone with a paper cup in front of you asking for money. If you left your apartment building and walked a block to go to the deli, there was a good chance you'd encounter someone seeking to separate you from your change as you came out with your sandwich. If you sat down on a bench, you'd feel the need to be looking out from both sides of your eyes for the arrival of an unwelcome solicitor. And certainly if you took a ride in a subway you'd think it odd if you *weren't* accosted by a hustler.

New Yorkers inevitably found that they had a personal decision to make: to give or not to give, that was the question. Was there actually any chance that the person asking for your change really needed that money to get his next meal? Some felt that if even one in a hundred was in that category, the ethical thing to do was to give something to anyone who asked. Others felt that giving handouts to beggars was contributing to their substance abuse problem that they themselves weren't confronting and therefore the ethical thing to do was *not* to give. This was quite a dilemma to many, including taxi drivers.

When I began driving a cab, I usually found myself giving a quarter to anyone who would come up to me. But as years went by and cynicism grew, I gradually realized that it would take Sherlock Holmes to be able to differentiate someone who was actually a down-on-his-luck victim from an outright hustler. And Sherlock had better have a lie detector. I had been fooled too many times.

There was the young woman, for instance, who came running up to my cab with a gasoline can in her hand late one night when I was waiting at a red light on Queens Boulevard. Telling me breathlessly that her car had run out of gas and that she was stranded and frightened, she asked me for a dollar with a sincerity in her voice that would have made Mother Teresa proud. I gave her the buck and felt I had done my good deed for the day. The next night I found myself at the same light and the same young woman came running up to my cab with the same gas can and the same story.

Using a similar out-of-gas angle with a creative flair, there was the time a car driven by a middle-aged man pulled up next to my cab while I was parked on Lexington Avenue on a break. Apologizing for the intrusion, the man called over to me and explained that his car was almost out of gas and, embarrassing as this was, would I be kind enough to help him out with a dollar or two so he could make it home to Westchester? I called back to him that I could indeed give him a dollar but, no offense, I'd like to come over and look at his gas gauge first.

He drove away.

About a year later, again on Lexington Avenue, the same man pulled over next to me and tried the same scam. This time I threatened to write down his license plate number and report him to the police.

He drove away faster.

So, like many New Yorkers, I became hardened to the outstretched hands and the bodies attached to them. I even began to consider the possibility that in New York City there was no such thing as a truly down and out person who just needed some help to get him on his feet again or even to get him a train ticket back home to the suburbs. Certain contrary facts had crept in.

How come, for example, with so many beggars out there on the streets, there were always about ten ads for taxi drivers in the help-wanted pages of the newspapers on any given day? How come, for that matter, did all the fleets have permanent 'DRIVERS WANTED' bumper stickers displayed on their cabs? How come the great majority of drivers were immigrants? Was there some kind of conspiracy keeping Americans out of the business?

What I found out was that the taxi industry in New York *never* has enough drivers, even though you can make a livable wage if you do it full time. But it's a very tough job and there are no benefits. And while there's certainly no conspiracy keeping Americans out of the industry, the job is far below the standards expected in most American labor situations and so the immigrants wind up being the only ones willing to do it.

So it was clear that even though taxi-driving jobs were available in abundance, great numbers of people, apparently able-bodied in most cases, preferred to be out on the streets asking for handouts. Knowing this, a new question kept knocking on the door of my universe: how much money could someone make by begging in New York City? I thought it was one of those things you could never know until I realized that I had a way of finding out.

The numbers man

There was a hustler I had seen regularly on the streets for virtually ten years, usually on 57th Street. He approached me so many times asking for spare change (and never getting any) that I eventually learned his name, Willie, and became familiar with his modus operandi. Willie approached as many cars as he could possibly get to before the red light would turn green, never wasting any time. He would simply say, 'Spare some change?' to each driver and the moment he saw that the driver wasn't going to give him anything, he would *jog* to the next car to ask the next driver for money.

He didn't bother with recriminations, scowls, apologies or jokes. He just moved as quickly as possible to the next potential customer. When the light turned green on the side of the street where he'd just worked (57th is a two-way street), he would jog to the other side to hustle the drivers over there who were then waiting at a red light of their own.

Willie had, I believe, discovered the secret to success in professional begging. And the secret is that it's not so much how pathetic you look, it's how many people you approach with your hand open that determines your income. Not that it doesn't hurt to look somewhat pathetic or deranged. Willie did. In the summer he wore a dirty t-shirt and in the winter he put on a torn overcoat on which, on close inspection, you could see that the tears had been made with a scissor. The point is that quantity is more important than quality in this enterprise. Some people will give and some people won't. The more 'will give' people you approach, the more money you make. It's a numbers game.

How much money can an industrious beggar make? I realized the key to knowing this was to know two simple facts: 1) I observed that Willie would get, on the average, at least one person to give him something for each change of the light. I think it would be fair to say that the minimum amount of money given would be a quarter. 2) The lights change approximately once every thirty seconds in New York City.

From these two facts we can determine Willie's minimum income. Assuming he worked a forty-hour week, if he got a quarter for every change of the light, that's fifty cents a minute. Fifty cents a minute would give him $30 per hour. Multiply that by an eight-hour work day and you've got $240 a day. For a five-day week, that's $1,200. And for a fifty-week year (we give him a two-week vacation), his minimum take-home is $60,000!

But that's a minimum number. The truth is that Willie usually got more than one driver to give him something for each change of the light. Sometimes three or four people would oblige him. And many gave more than a quarter. I would often see a dollar bill finding its way into Willie's hands. Plus he worked more than eight hours a day. It wasn't unusual to see him at the beginning and at the end of my shift, and my shift goes for twelve hours.

So it would be safe to assume that Willie was actually making at least double the $60,000 figure – $120,000 – and I think even that is a low number. In any case, I believe it's more than what the mayor was being paid in those days.

*

So you see how easy it was for me to become more than a little cynical on the subject of people coming up to me asking for a handout. And my cynicism only worsened by learning some inside information one day from a certain passenger in my cab…

The human garbage bag

One evening in October, 1997, I was driving a middle-aged man from Midtown to the Upper East Side when the silence of our ride was interrupted by a young man coming up to the side of the cab asking for money. As you already know, I am not a likely candidate for a handout, especially when the seeker is considerably younger than me, and this guy got zilch. However, his presence led to a conversation between me and my passenger about the situation with hustlers in the city. I made some comment to him about not being able to tell the difference between actual victims and outright hustlers nor even between actual substance abusers and outright hustlers, and this brought a response from him that, as a police officer, he has often had the same problem. He had come into contact with lots of hustlers over the years and remarked that they were often ingenious in being able to appear as something other than what they really were.

A police officer! Aha! I realized I had a rare opportunity on my hands. Whenever I've seen beggars on the street I've always wondered what their story was. How did they come to this? Were they for real? But I knew I could never find out. Even if I asked one of them to tell me, I probably wouldn't believe whatever story he'd dish out anyway because I'd figure it was part of the hustle.

But a police officer dealing with people like this would have a chance of knowing what the truth was. If a hustler was hauled down to the precinct on a loitering or public nuisance charge, the cops could detain him until his actual identity was established. And then they might be able to find out what was actually going on with this person.

So I asked my passenger this question: who was his favorite hustler of all time? He thought about it for just a few moments and then a smile lit up his face. And he told me the story of The Human Garbage Bag. As he began speaking I realized that I knew exactly whom he was talking about. I had seen this person on the streets myself many times.

The Human Garbage Bag was a forty-something woman who appeared on the streets in cold weather wearing nothing but a torn-up pair of shoes and a plastic, green garbage bag, the kind you see piled up on the sidewalk waiting for the arrival of the Sanitation Department. She was about five-foot-one, dark-skinned, and quite thin, even gaunt. The garbage bag fit snugly around her body, the top of it just covering her breasts and the bottom curving around her buttocks, leaving her shoulders, most of her back and her legs exposed to the weather. Her hair was a frazzled mess, flying off in all directions, and she always had a dazed, far-away look in her eyes, as if lack of food and exposure to the elements had rendered her partially demented. I remembered that whenever I had seen her on the street her condition had drawn my attention to the plight of the homeless and made me feel a little guilty that I had it so good as a taxi driver. I would find myself wondering what the hell we were coming to as a society, anyway.

But here is her real story (and again I reiterate how extraordinary it is to have learned this, since this kind of information is never, *never* able to be gotten a hold of, unless you're a cop or God): she was a professional actress.

My passenger told me she had studied in some of the best acting schools and performed many times on the stage. She lived in a $400,000 house in Westchester County and had three children. She traveled into the city in a van which she parked on the street and used as her dressing room. Here she changed into her costume (the garbage bag) and added whatever cosmetic touches were helpful to further create her character. He went on to tell me that during the Christmas season people would actually *wait in line* to give her money and that she could take in as much as $4,000 in a single day!

Now I don't want to diminish the problems of people who are truly down and out or give you the impression that I'm so cynical that I think *everyone* who comes up to you asking for money is a fake. Surely there are great numbers of true, hopeless-case, haven't-been-sober-in-a-year derelicts out there.

Like *this* guy…

On the Bowery

The Bowery is an avenue in lower Manhattan that runs from Chinatown to the East Village, then changes its name to 3rd Avenue. Due to the fact that for so many years large contingents of derelicts could be found there, 'on the Bowery' as a phrase became synonymous in the language with being a bum.

'Whatever happened to John?' someone might have asked.

'John? Oh, poor John, he's on the Bowery,' might have been the sad answer, meaning not that John was literally on the Bowery but that John was an alcoholic who could no longer function in society. By the '90s the Bowery itself and the areas around it began to change into a much more upscale neighborhood, but prior to that a cab driver knew what to expect whenever he drove there.

There was one intersection in particular, Houston Street and the Bowery, where as surely as spring follows winter, thunder follows lightning, and indigestion follows pepperoni, you would find upon stopping there at any time of night or day that a derelict was coming toward you to present his case for why giving him money for his next bottle of booze was the right thing to do.

Being fully aware of this fact and not liking these encounters with bums, I always tried to avoid stopping at Houston and the

Bowery. But a force greater than our own seems to have decreed that from whatever direction you approach it, you will always hit a red light at that intersection. And that's exactly what happened one sunny day in November, 1980, as I was heading east on Houston with two passengers in the back.

Without even bothering to look around, I automatically warned them that they should be prepared for an onslaught of alcoholics. It was that predictable. But, oddly enough, no one approached us. In fact, by some twist of fate, there wasn't a derelict anywhere in sight other than an unshaven, white-haired man who was sitting with his back resting against a lamppost in the middle of the concrete median that separates the two directions of traffic on Houston Street. He held a sandwich in his hand and stared vacantly ahead, completely minding his own business.

Relieved, I mentioned to my passengers how fortunate we were. Being familiar with this part of the city, they agreed that it was indeed unusual not to be harassed at this intersection, and they then resumed their conversation, which as I recall concerned the value of the dollar against other currencies.

I had nothing to do but wait for the light to turn green and found myself gazing aimlessly around at the environment, my attention eventually becoming fixed on this bum sitting against the lamppost. He was still eating his sandwich and was apparently oblivious to everything around him when he suddenly turned his head and looked straight at me, catching me staring at him. As our eyes locked, I realized he was about to speak. I braced myself for the inevitable plea for money and I'd already decided that he wouldn't get a dime out of me.

And then he spoke:

'Don't bother me now,' he said, *'I'm on my lunch break.'*

A question of responsibility

I had just come across the Manhattan Bridge from Brooklyn on a June night in 1979 and was heading uptown when I once again found myself stopped at the red light at Houston and the Bowery. As if on cue, a figure emerged from the shadows and slowly lumbered toward me.

He was a bum's bum. The uneven walk, the half-closed eyes and the filthy belly sticking out from under his filthy shirt would tell even the most obtuse passerby that here was a career derelict, a truly hopeless case.

I tried to wave him off but, of course, it was to no avail. He slumped over across the hood of my cab and began to wipe the windshield with his hand – no greasy towel, just his hand. After a couple of token wipes he pulled himself off the hood and stood motionlessly beside me at the side of the taxi, his palm turned up in anticipation of the hoped-for dime or quarter and his eyes gazing vacantly into the farthest reaches of intoxicated space.

I will admit that in my early years of taxi-driving I had something of a morally indignant attitude when it came to drunks. So I thought I would enlighten him and therefore change his life forever by posing a question to him.

'If you can correctly answer one simple question,' I said, 'I'll give you a dollar.'

He started to become a bit more alert, as if awakening from a long sleep.

'Who is responsible for the condition you're in?' I asked.

I'd never seen a man's demeanor change so quickly. His eyes regained their focus and he smiled broadly, revealing a set of crooked teeth that hadn't been brushed for three years. He answered my question without hesitation, and he answered it with the enthusiasm of a contestant on a quiz show who was absolutely certain he was about to win the jackpot.

'I AM!' he cried out.

He got the dollar. And I got a little life lesson: that what drives a human being to dereliction cannot in the slightest way be solved by a condescending question posed by a taxi driver.

Zak

What can be so disturbing and even depressing about encounters with those whom you know for sure are really hardcore substance abusers and not merely scam artists is the hopelessness they emit. A natural human desire to help them is triggered by these meetings which is quickly snuffed out by the realization that you cannot. Then added to that is the thought that they surely don't have much time to live, for who could go on for very long existing the way that they do? Begging for handouts so you can get your next bottle of booze is the last stop on the line, brother.

So a certain passenger I had in my cab one night in April, 1983 turned out to be something of an inspiration to me when I heard his story. He was an oddball – I could see that at a glance – but a harmless one, eager to talk about anything in general and himself in particular. There was a distinct wildness behind his eyes, as if his mind were an animal that had not quite been domesticated.

His name was Zak, he said, and he worked as a dishwasher now, although his true calling was that of an artist, a painter. But he had formerly been a Bowery bum.

Zak carried with him some photographs of his paintings and showed me two of them. They were kind of mystical in nature with lots of moons, strange symbols and long-haired women. I thought they weren't half bad. What interested me most, however, was his former existence as a derelict. 'Former' Bowery bums are a rarity, indeed.

He'd spent two years on the Bowery, he said, a two-year drunk sleeping in doorways or flophouses and panhandling with 'the boys'. He'd never been able to stick with a career or a wife and was spending his life working menial jobs in different cities. He'd run up a number of sizable gambling debts that he couldn't pay and which appeared to give him no option but to hit the road and hope that the bookies or their goons never caught up with him. Eventually he arrived in New York, a city big enough to disappear into, and the Bowery seemed the logical place to go. And for two years it was home.

Zak's lucky break was that somehow something clicked internally that rehabilitated a purpose for living, and that purpose was his art. Then, with the help of the Salvation Army, he was able to step away from and overcome his cravings for alcohol. He'd been sober for five years.

What, I wanted to know, had become of the guys he used to hang around with on the Bowery?

'Everyone I knew,' Zak said, 'is dead.'

Without a leg to stand on

So you see that these continual encounters with beggars had created some ambivalence in me. The story of Zak changed my point of view for a while and I began again to give coins to those who looked like there might be at least some chance that they weren't outright hustlers. But as time went on my compassion waned and I closed shop. I became numb to the endless parade and my thinking fell into line with: real change comes from within, why don't you get a job, don't take me for an idiot, and who do I look like, Santa Claus?

Nobody got a dime.

And with that policy firmly in place, I pulled up to a red light behind three other cars at the intersection of 23rd Street and 11th Avenue on a sunny day in May, 1988. A woman in a wheelchair suddenly appeared from the sidewalk and pushed herself in the direction of the first car.

The thought that came immediately to mind was that she was probably as fleet-footed as a gazelle and that the wheelchair was just a prop to gain sympathy and cash. Here was yet another creative hustler who had invested in a money machine, the wheelchair, and probably made more cabbage in two hours than I did in a day. But as she got a little closer I saw that I was wrong, at least about the fleet-footed part, because this woman had no feet. In fact, she had no legs.

There was no faking it. It was clear that both her legs had been amputated at the knees, the stumps fully visible because she had rolled her shorts up as high as they could go to the tops of her thighs. Her face was reddened from a combination of alcohol consumption and exposure to the weather and her hair was matted in clumps. She was, in fact, the very embodiment of a human train wreck.

The drivers of the cars in front of me each gave something to the woman, but I was unmoved in my viewpoint. There was plenty of help available to well-meaning people who had lost limbs, I reasoned. Why couldn't she avail herself of it instead of making herself out to be an object of pity? I quickly decided that, legs or no legs, she was no different than any other hustler and she would get not a farthing out of me. In fact, as she rolled up to my cab I was even thinking of saying something sarcastic to her like, 'Can you give me some advice on how to invest my disposable income?' Or, 'Do you vacation in the Caribbean or the Virgin Islands?' Or, 'Do you own my apartment building? You look just like my landlord.'

But then, as she came up right beside me, I saw that her condition was far worse than the fact that her legs had been amputated. On her stumps were open sores, disgusting red welts that were oozing out white liquid pus.

I thought I was beyond being shocked by anything I could see on the streets of New York, but this did the trick. My defenses shattered, I found myself reaching for a dollar and handing it to her through the window, something I thought I might never again do. She took the bill and said 'thank you' in a voice that was a carrier wave for all the sorrows that have ever existed in this world.

As the light turned green and I proceeded toward 10th Avenue, I found myself shook up mentally by what had just happened. I felt I'd done the right thing by giving her something, but I was upset with myself for how cold and callous my initial intentions had been. The very thought that I had been considering saying something cruel to this pitiful wretch disturbed me deeply. How did I become one of the heartless people that I myself don't like? Had I been in New York City too long? How the hell did I ever get to be this cynical?

As I pulled up to another red light at 10th, I continued to spin in my introspection. I almost didn't notice the rear door open and a passenger get in.

'Penn Station,' his voice said.

I snapped into present time. It was good to have a passenger just now. I most definitely needed someone to talk to, and I told him about the woman with no legs and how pathetic she was.

'Oh, yeah,' he said, 'she's been out there for years.'

'She *has*? How do you know?'

'My apartment is right there across the street,' he replied cheerfully. 'I see her all the time. She has prosthetic legs under the wheelchair. She puts them on at the end of the day and pushes the wheelchair home.'

'She *does*? But she has all these horrible sores all over her stumps. What about *that*?'

He actually started to laugh.

'Right,' he said, 'she paints them on with make-up. I've watched her do it from my window. Amazing, huh?'

Well, that handled my introspection. I now understood that after all these years of driving a cab my problem wasn't that I was *too* cynical. My problem was that *I wasn't cynical enough*!

Damn!

*

I will admit, however, that hustlers, although they may never again get anything from me but a smile, do make up one of the elements of New York that give it its gritty charm. And I've never felt that they should all be rounded up and shipped off to the frontier, as I do the people who are the subject of the next chapter of this book.

9

Pedestrians

In New York City we have a certain segment of the population who think nothing of risking their lives just to avoid the annoyance of having to wait fifteen seconds for a light to turn green. So confident are these maniacs of their own agility and timing that they will allow the eager hands of Death to come within an inch of yanking them over to the Other Side before they would consider actually moving out of the way. We have a special name for these people. No, it's not 'stuntmen' or 'daredevils'. We call them 'pedestrians'.

Here's a joke I've told a million times: a passenger gets in the back seat and asks me how long I've been driving a cab.

'Since 1977,' I say, 'and I've never hit a pedestrian.'

'Well, thank goodness for that!' the passenger replies.

'No, no, you don't understand,' I protest, 'it isn't that I haven't *tried!* Every time I think I've got one they slip out of the way at the last second! They're like pigeons!'

Crossing the street in New York is a 'see it, go for it' affair. There's no such thing as enforcement of jaywalking laws, and the 'walk – don't walk' signal is merely the wishful thinking of some civic-minded do-gooder who *must* have been kidding. In fact, if you see someone actually standing on the sidewalk waiting for the 'walk' signal to appear when there are no cars around, it looks odd. Probably a tourist or a police cadet.

I will confess that, although I take special effort to avoid speaking in generalities, pedestrians are the one segment of the human race that I disdain as a group. Think about it – what good are pedestrians to a taxi driver? For one thing, every one of them is a potential lawsuit if the side of your cab should so much as rub up against their precious little leg. For another thing, they're clogging up the intersections, preventing *me* from getting where *I* want to go. And for one more thing, they're walking instead of riding, and that's bad for business, mister.

I've always found it amusing, by the way, when passengers get in the cab and kind of apologize for taking a ride that's so short that they could have walked it. I remind them that, hey, I don't make any money if you walk, so there's no need to apologize to *me*, and I will also point out some of the dangers of walking that they may not have considered:

- You could get hit on the head by an air conditioner falling out of a window.
- You could get hit, for that matter, by a meteorite.
- You could meet someone on the street whom you've been trying to avoid.
- You could be electrocuted by stepping on a metal plate (it has happened).
- You could suffer public humiliation by getting your heel stuck in a grating.
- You could slip on a banana peel (it happens in cartoons all the

time, right?).

- And, worst of all, you could step on a crack and break your mother's back.

But regardless of my warnings, people keep walking in New York City in huge numbers. I've had ample opportunity to observe them and I have concluded that pedestrians can be categorized into these basic types:

1. The Get To Live Another Day People

2. The Dare-yas

3. The One Inch Wonders

4. The Oblivious

5. The Immortals

Let's examine them one by one, but, before we do, I would like to point out that no matter which category a pedestrian fits into, what's going on in the street is basically a struggle for possession of territory. In a city with limited space but unlimited people (and dogs) it often appears that someone else is in the place where *you* want to be. Hence, the conflict. It's how a person operates within this struggle that puts him into a category.

First, it should be said that not *everyone* is daring Fate. Most New Yorkers *do* walk – or run – cautiously, and they are the Get To Live Another Day People. They may take longer to get to where they're going, but they do get to live and procreate the species. And now that this has been duly noted, let's move on. The Get

To Live Another Day People are alive but they're boring.

Now, have you ever witnessed this? A car is waiting at a red light at an intersection and pedestrians are walking in front of that car from one side of the street to the other. The signal starts flashing 'don't walk', but several pedestrians keep coming anyway. Finally the light turns green for the car that's been sitting there, but, wait, one more pedestrian comes along and crosses by in front of the car. Then, just as the car begins to accelerate, *another* pedestrian suddenly comes briskly walking or even jogging right into the path of the vehicle. This pedestrian gives no sign of flinching or stopping, he just keeps moving forward, causing the car to either hit the brakes or hit him. The car, of course, stops. That's a Dare-ya.

The unspoken sentiment here is, 'This is *my* territory, pal. This little strip of asphalt here? That's *mine.* Come on, hit me. Make my day. I *dare ya.*' A variant on this is the Double Dare-ya, which is when someone does the same thing but instead of moving quickly, he *saunters* in front of the vehicle, usually while on his cell phone or talking with his friends who are coming up just behind him. Utterly maddening to a taxi driver.

Taking it one step further (pun intended), a Triple Dare-ya actually *stops walking* right in front of your car. He may decide that this is the place where he's going to light his cigarette or adjust his backpack. There have been cases reported in which Triple Dare-yas have been rumored to have kneeled over and tied their shoelaces right in front of yellow cabs in New York City, but I have never personally witnessed such an outrage.

One of the dangers of an encounter with a Dare-ya is the potential for conflict. If you hit your brakes too hard or start moving the vehicle too soon, even if nothing was meant by it, a Dare-ya having a bad hair day may strike back. The lowest gradient of this is the disapproving glance. Then there is the 'stare down', in which the Dare-ya stops in his tracks and gives you the evil eye. You resist the impulse of returning your foot to the accelerator and finishing the job.

These confrontations can get ugly. One can be flipped the bird, one can be compared to an aperture at the very end of the alimentary canal, and, worse still, the gradient can shoot right out the top into some sort of sudden street violence. I have numerous times been reminded that I came too close by hearing a thud from somebody's hand against the side of my cab as I kept driving by. I have had my windshield receive an unwanted spit bath. And I once witnessed a driver, who had rolled up his window in an attempt to block out a barrage of insults, have that window smashed to bits by the fist of an enraged Dare-ya.

Child sacrifice

I picked up a passenger one evening around 9 a.m. at 60th Street and 5th Avenue who was heading down to Penn Station at 34th and 7th. The traffic by this time of the night thins out considerably and so it becomes possible to ride the wave of green lights down 5th in order to get the passenger to his train really quickly. The strategy is to avoid the congestion of Times Square by staying on 5th until you're south of 42nd Street, and only then cutting across to 7th Avenue. I usually choose 37th Street as my cross-town route.

Now, if you are near the front of the wave as you go down 5th, and you make the right turn on 37th, you can make the green light at the next intersection, 6th Avenue, if you step on it just a bit. Fortunately for the passenger, who had only seven minutes to make his train, there were no vehicles whatsoever on 37th Street, so making that green at 6th was a sure thing if I could keep moving. I brought my speed up to thirty miles per hour (the limit in Manhattan) and I could see ahead that, since no other cars were on the street, a steady stream of pedestrians were crossing against the light in the intersection. Knowing that since they were New Yorkers they were going to keep walking until I was right on top of them, and knowing also that I needed to maintain my speed in order to make the light, I sounded the horn when I was about seventy-five yards from the light to give notice that I was *comin' through.*

Most human beings in this situation would know two things without even thinking about it:

1. That, since their signal says 'don't walk', they do *not* have the right of way, and

2. That, right of way or no right of way, there is a goddamned taxicab barreling down the street at you and even if you move out of the way at the last millisecond, you better freaking do it, Charlie.

Enter the Dare-ya.

It was a heavyset woman in a bomber jacket. Ignoring the rightness or wrongness of the situation, a deeper, gut-level instinct cut in and told her that her territorial rights were senior to the laws of taxi drivers and physics. *She* was the immoveable object, not the puny taxicab. She would make her stand here on the sacred tarmac of 37th and 6th, and, as God is her witness, she would never – *never!* – be forced off her land again.

So she stopped in the middle of the intersection, turned, and stared me down, clearly showing the Lord above and the pedestrians below that she was willing to give her life for The Cause.

Oh, and one other thing – not only was she willing to give *her* life, she was also willing to sacrifice the life of the little child she was holding by the hand.

I hit the brakes. I stopped. The light turned yellow. The light turned red. The woman stood her ground in the middle of the intersection and glared at me like a wildebeest confronting a leopard. I glared back at her like a cab driver confronting a lunatic. And then the screaming began. Whatever curses she shot at me and my ancestors could not be deciphered due to my not being able to hear them over the curses *I* was machine-gunning at her and *her* ancestors. Thirty seconds of this, then the light turned green and I continued on my way, wishing once again that I was a cop.

I still got the guy to Penn Station on time.

More common than the Dare-ya is the One Inch Wonder. The One Inch Wonder will walk against the light and will stop his motion to let you go by – but only by an inch. You'll see him zigging and zagging his way across an avenue filled with oncoming vehicles like a matador tip-toeing around *el toro*. The agility, the balance and the prediction of motion of an oncoming object could be viewed as an urban aesthetic performance, if not a tourist attraction. It's quite a marvel to behold.

Here's an example that I see every day. The one-way avenues in Manhattan are timed so that if you go about twenty-seven miles per hour, you will never hit a red light unless you're slowed down by traffic. This is the 'wave' that I just mentioned. Quite often when the evening rush hours are finished and the traffic has thinned out, only a few vehicles will be moving along together at the front of the wave and behind them will be a handful of straggling cars bringing up the rear. Rather than stay back at a safe distance until the last car has passed by, the One Inch Wonders will start to cross the avenue against the light and give the approaching vehicles just the slightest bit of room – an inch! – in which to pass. The assumption is that none of the cars will suddenly veer to the left or right and run them down. The amazing idiocy here is that the One Inch Wonder is risking all – literally his very life or at least his life without paralysis or broken bones – in order to gain a few seconds of not-standing-still-time.

There's a cure, by the way, for the antics of the One Inch Wonders and for the defiance of the Dare-yas, too – something that's sure to make a better pedestrian out of anybody. And that is to be an eyewitness to someone being hit by a car. Most people living in large cities have at one time or another seen the aftermath of it, but few have actually witnessed the impact itself. I have seen it four times. And I want you to know, it gives you a healthy respect for the physics involved in car versus the human body. It's a sickening sight, even at a relatively slow speed.

Which brings us to the Oblivious. According to recent statistics, about three hundred people die each year in traffic accidents in New York City, and half of them are pedestrians who are hit by vehicles. I suspect that the majority are not Dare-yas or One Inch Wonders, but people who are just not paying attention – the Oblivious. It's easy to fall into this category in New York, where there's so much going on. Somebody walking six dogs on six leashes – head turns. Sudden aroma of roasted garlic permeating the air – head turns. Girl comes along wearing almost nothing but a bikini, entire body does a one-eighty. Add to this the popularity of listening to iPods, chattering on cell phones, and texting while walking and you may conclude that it's surprising that more people aren't run over. Actually, it *is* surprising.

In a subsection of this category are the Sheep, who are oblivious in their own particular way. Instead of having their attention yanked away from them by distractions in the environment, they have blanked out everything but their own universe except for the movement of the people right in front of them, whom they follow blindly. Their troubles begin when the person in front of them turns out to be a One Inch Wonder.

If not run over by a truck, the Oblivious can often be found stranded in the middle of an avenue with cars whizzing around them on all sides. This is an urban sideshow and what has always amazed me about it is the inevitable moronic smile on the face of the humiliated wanderer. Death approaching on all sides, and there's always that dumb-ass-me grin. However, not everyone who finds himself in the middle of an avenue filled with oncoming vehicles is an Oblivious. There's one other category which can be difficult to spot, but if you look carefully you will see them – the Immortals!

A race of superhuman beings living on the island of Manhattan, the Immortals mingle in with the population of ordinary people and can go completely unobserved unless you know what to look for. We're not certain where they come from or exactly what powers they may possess, but we do know one thing about them for sure: they cannot be killed, harmed or injured in any way. If you grabbed one of them and threw him from the top of a ten-story building, somehow there would be a truck full of feathers waiting for him at the bottom.

I'm sure you've seen some of them occasionally if you've spent any time at all in Manhattan. You just didn't know what you were looking at. How can you tell? They will be performing some daredevil act with such utter disregard for their own safety that you'll think they're out of touch with reality. They can be confused with the Oblivious but the test is how they react when the eighteen-wheeler swerves at the last second to avoid flattening them into a potato chip. The Oblivious will have a holy-shit-I-can't-believe-I'm-still-alive response. The Immortals will not bat an eye, which actually demonstrates the fact that they are very much in touch with reality. And that reality is that they are Immortals and cannot be scratched.

Here's a common example: with cars and trucks whizzing down an avenue, all doing around thirty-five miles per hour, an Immortal begins his excursion from one side of that avenue to the other. He doesn't lift his head to make eye contact with the drivers nor does he zig and zag as vehicles come oh so very close. He just keeps his head down, too involved in the more important machinations of his innermost world, and continues walking, unscathed and unconcerned, to the other side.

That is an Immortal.

Here's another example: you are strolling along on a sidewalk in Manhattan and you hear some vile language being used. You look around and are shocked to see that there's someone shouting obscenities right into the face of a cop. The cop just stands there, maybe even smiles. This goes on for a minute or so and then the person calmly walks away.

That is an Immortal.

If you or I were to attempt these stunts, we would last about twenty seconds. But to an Immortal, it's all in a day's work.

Touchy bastard

I was driving down 2nd Avenue with a passenger in my cab one October evening in 1986 at about nine o'clock. The weather was crisp and clear and the vehicles around me on the avenue were moving rapidly. As we approached 66th Street I spotted something about a block down the road that caused me great alarm: it was a blind old man with a cane who was trying to make his way across 2nd Avenue while cars kept zipping by all around him. He was coming perilously close to being run over and none of the other drivers had the decency to stop for a few moments so he could make it safely across to the other side. I made an instant decision that I was going to do something about it, even if no one else gave a damn.

'I've got to help this guy,' I said to my passenger, a woman who was trying to get to Grand Central, and I brought my cab to an abrupt halt right next to the old man in the middle of the avenue. My passenger was okay with this, offering support and warning me to be careful as I opened my door in the midst of the traffic.

With some disregard for my own safety, I jumped out, held my arms above my head, and walked out in front of a lane of oncoming vehicles, ordering (yes, *ordering*) them to stop. The cars and trucks in that lane all came to an immediate halt. Excellent! I then confronted the next lane in the same manner and brought them to a stop, too.

The way was now cleared for the blind man to walk safely to the other side, and if I don't say so myself, I was nothing short of magnificent! I had already decided that I was a hero and half-expected to see people leaning out of their windows on 2nd Avenue, cheering me on and waving little flags. Maybe some tourists had witnessed my daring act and would go back to Kansas City to tell their friends that New Yorkers weren't so cold and uncaring after all.

I reached out to the blind man and said, 'Come with me, sir.' He had an immediate reaction as he felt my hand touch his arm:

'Keep your hands off of me, you fucking idiot!' he screamed, and then he started swinging his cane wildly in the air to drive me away from him.

I stood there dumbfounded, staring stupidly at him until he finished walking to the sidewalk. By that time all the vehicles which I'd so brilliantly brought to a halt started moving again in unison and now *I* was the one stuck in the middle of 2nd Avenue!

I was lucky to make it back to my cab alive and could barely be consoled by my passenger's acknowledgment that it was a good thing to do even if the old man turned out to be a jerk. After finishing my shift in a state of deep introspection, wondering where it had all gone wrong, I had a realization about what had happened. It was just that this guy was an Immortal. What else could explain it?

Although we don't know much about them, we could assume that their preoccupation with their own thoughts must make the mundane affairs of humans intolerable. Hell, nobody says that just because you're an Immortal you have to be a nice guy. Quite the opposite appears to be true. Actually, when you get right down to it, they're touchy bastards.

*

So inasmuch as I would like to see pedestrians completely banished from the streets of New York, I have to admit that it appears likely that they are here to stay. If you should find yourself joining their ranks, let me warn you (and I say this seriously) that the most dangerous thing in the Monster City of the World is not being mugged by a thug or getting drunk and then finding that you no longer have any shoes and there's a tattoo on your neck – it is getting to the other side of the street in one piece.

Knowing his limits

I picked up a young man in June, 1999 who asked me for an odd piece of information. He wanted to know if I could tell him how high the Empire State Building was. I told him I thought it was eighty-six stories, not counting the upper observation deck and the tower, but what he wanted to know was if I knew its measurement in terms of feet or meters, which I did not. Since this was such a weird thing to ask a cab driver, I naturally was curious to find out why he would want to know it. His answer got my attention.

He said he was thinking of jumping off the Empire State Building with a parachute and didn't yet know if there was enough distance from the top of the building to the ground to enable his chute to open up in time. It was a project that was still in the planning stages.

Oh. Of course. Why didn't I think of that?

Well, it wasn't going to be difficult to have a conversation with this fellow. I soon learned the whole story. He was about twenty-five years old, an American by birth, but had spent most of his childhood in Holland. Somewhere in his teens he had taken up the sport of skydiving and was now, in my words, a thrill-seeking junkie. But it wasn't just for thrills, actually, it was also for profit.

His idea was to jump off the Empire State Building while his friends videotaped him from the ground, escape in a van, and then sell the footage to television producers.

I told him I didn't think he could get past security with a parachute in the Empire State Building. Although this was prior to 9/11, about a year earlier a maniac had gone up to the Observation Deck with a gun and had opened fire, killing one tourist and injuring several others before shooting himself. I assumed security had been pretty tight after that. Besides, I said, why would he want to do anything so ridiculously dangerous? Isn't it good to be alive?

His response to my concern was interesting to me. He said it wasn't dangerous if you had done your research and knew what you were doing as a skydiver. You needed a certain amount of clearance from the point from which you'd jumped and you needed a certain amount of distance for the parachute to be able to open to its full capacity. If you knew these things without any chance of miscalculation, it was not dangerous, at least according to him.

But what about landing on the street, I wanted to know. How could he be sure he wouldn't come down in front of a truck on 5th Avenue? For that matter, how could he be sure the wind wouldn't pick up and carry him across town into the river or into electric wires somewhere? He told me that skydivers can control the direction of their descent with steering devices that are a part of the parachute.

'I can put myself down between two lanes of traffic,' he said, 'it's not a problem.' This was something I didn't know. It explained how skydiving stunts are performed, things like parachutists jumping out of planes and coming down in the middle of a football field. I was impressed.

The thing that did concern him, however, had nothing to do with safety. It had to do with the regulations that govern the world of skydiving. You need to have a license to be a skydiver. If you get caught pulling off an illegal stunt, you will lose your license. That would mean that you wouldn't be able to jump out of planes anymore because any pilot who would allow an unlicensed skydiver to leap from his aircraft would in turn lose his own license. That's the way the sport is controlled and it was the only concern of my passenger, not his safety.

Since I am rather fearful of heights, the idea that someone could jump from an extreme elevation and not have concerns about its danger was amazing to me. But I'm thinking everyone is afraid of *something*, right? So I asked him this brilliant question:

'Tell me something,' I said, 'if you don't think jumping off the Empire State Building is dangerous, what *do* you think is dangerous?'

He thought about it for a few moments. And then he said these words, and he said them with a straight face and without any attempt at humor:

'Crossing the street against the light.'

Jump off the Empire State Building?

Sure.

Cross the street against the light?

What do you think I am? *Crazy???*

10

Road Rage

As irritating as pedestrians may be to a cabbie, they are mere inconveniences when compared to the real conflict that is always in progress on the streets of New York: the endless struggle between taxi driver and every other vehicle on the road for possession of space. Trying to make the light before it turns red? There's a minivan from New Jersey in front of you going ten miles per hour. Want to pull into your favorite taxi stand so you can get a coffee and enjoy a civilized piss? Sorry, police cars have decided the stand now belongs to them. Think you can get to that woman who's trying to hail a cab up on the next block? No, a rental truck with Colorado plates blocks your way and another taxi gets to her first.

You are entering here a world of desire, greed, speed, sloth, idiocy, misunderstood intentions, arrogance, ignorance, blind spots and obscene hand gestures. It's the world of road rage and it's nasty.

You would probably think at first glance that the madhouse streets of New York would almost automatically make for a situation of perpetual road rage for anyone who had to be out there all the time making a living in it. Most passengers who ask me what it is that drives me the craziest about driving a cab think it's the traffic, but it's not. Actually, after about six months a taxi driver builds up a tolerance to traffic, kind of like an immunity. It slides off your back. I call this the 'hump'. If a cabbie can't get over the hump, he'd better find himself a new occupation, for he will surely go mad.

Nevertheless, even with this tolerance in place, road rage incidents do occur. But it takes something special, something so particularly outrageous that the impulse to react is irresistible. After long years of observation, I have concluded that these incidents can be placed into two general categories: a) road rage with 'civilians' and b) road rage with professionals.

By 'civilians' I mean drivers who aren't doing it for a living. Professionals include not only taxi drivers, but bus drivers, truck drivers, those pedicab guys and even the drivers of horse-drawn carriages. Not included in this category are the drivers of police cars, ambulances and fire trucks because there is no such thing as a road rage incident with them. When it comes to the roads, they are the elite. They've got sirens and flashing lights and it is understood by one and all that you just get out of their way. Of course.

Of the two categories, civilians are the more delicate particle. You've got to be careful with these guys. Road rage incidents may flare up suddenly and unexpectedly with civilians because they may not be used to the assertive style of driving that is normal in New York City. You cut off some guy in a souped-up Camaro who thinks he's the king of the road and you may see that Camaro speed up and attempt to run you off of that road. Do the same thing to another cabbie or a bus driver and it's hardly noticed. Also the civilian is more likely to flip out simply because he's not on the job. Anyone who's driving for a living may have his livelihood endangered by his failure to put the brakes on his own temper.

But be they professionals or civilians, there is one form of communication that is more likely than any other to perpetuate fury on the street. One little gesture, hardly threatening in a physical sense, but it packs the explosive power of a hand grenade. Ladies and gentlemen, introducing the star of road rage… *the finger*!

There can be no doubt that road rage incidents would reduce to nearly zero if people could only be born without their middle fingers. Actually, it's rather odd, if you think about it, that raising a particular digit into the air should provoke such passion. Raise your index finger up and people think you're pointing at something. Raise your thumb up and they think you love them. But raise that middle finger up… oh my God, it's war.

Having witnessed too many times what a reckless finger can do, I maintain a personal policy of never flipping the bird no matter how completely justified it would be to do so. And, conversely, I hold to the rule of always turning the other palm when it's flipped at me. But there are times when my mental off-switch is not quite as fast as my digital on-switch. Up goes the finger, and on comes the trouble.

Slow motion bird

I was heading back to Manhattan late one night from Brooklyn and just before making a right turn from Atlantic Avenue onto Boerum Place, the road that leads directly onto the Brooklyn Bridge, there was a welcome sight standing just off the curb: three wholesome-looking twenty-somethings with their hands in the air, indicating they were in need of my services. I stopped the cab and they began to climb in, a process which, with three of them, would take about fifteen seconds.

The driver of the car just behind me, a faceless man in a mid-sized black sedan, was less than pleased. His motion had been stopped and now he would have to suffer through fifteen seconds of not moving when he wanted to be moving. He decided to express his outrage by sounding his horn. Not a tap, nor even a tap-tap-tap. It was a full-frontal, uninterrupted torrent of noise that would presumably continue until the three of them were in the cab and we were in motion once again.

I did a one-second mental review of what had just happened. I was in the lane of traffic just a few inches from the curb, so I hadn't stopped for the passengers illegally or awkwardly. I hadn't jumped across from another lane to get to them, so I hadn't cut the guy off. I hadn't braked hard, causing him to brake hard himself. In fact, I had done absolutely nothing to warrant being honked at. I was simply stopping for passengers who wanted a taxi exactly the way I'm supposed to do. And to make it worse, at this particular intersection there was a sign that tells drivers that it's okay to make a right turn on a red, a rarity in New York City. So I wasn't even preventing him from making the light.

The conclusion flashed across my mind that the guy was beyond rude. He was evil. Now, this should have been the reason *not* to do what I then did, but stimulus–response got the best of me. I reached for the bird.

Out went my left hand through the window. Up came the finger. But instead of the usual jab into the sky and then a quick retreat, I executed the maneuver in slow motion, Statue of Liberty-style, with my arm coming to a full stop at its maximum length for a few seconds, topped off by a little wag of Mister Fuck You. This was repeated several times, a little quicker with each repetition, until my three passengers had entered the taxi and closed the door. With his horn still screeching, we were on our way.

Immediately, *middle finger regret* set in. Considering how angry the nut job already was to begin with for who-knows-why, I knew I'd been unwise to exacerbate the situation. Retaliation was now a certainty but I didn't know exactly what form it would take. For all I knew, he might pull out a gun. It seemed within the realm of possibility. So I prepared for whatever was to come as best I could. After instructing my passengers to 'hold on', I watched the guy carefully in my mirrors. I had taken the left lane on the three-lane Boerum Place after making the right from Atlantic and stepped on the gas in the hope of making the bridge without Mr Lunatic catching up to us. He had taken the middle lane and was gaining on me and I realized that no matter how fast I drove, he was determined to catch up to me and 'even the score'. I didn't want to drive so fast that my own speed would be more of a danger than he was, so I decided on a strategy that was right out of an action movie.

Instead of continuing to gain speed, I held steady at about sixty miles per hour and let the guy pull up even with me on the right side. Then, just as he passed me, he did what I expected him to do: he cut right in front of me and started to hit his brakes hard in an attempt to make me either crash into him or bring me to a halt. It was an insane action but – guess what? – the guy was insane. Being prepared for his move, I made a move of my own of braking harder than he did just as he got in front of me and then swerving violently around him into the far-right lane. I then stepped on the gas and opened it up, hoping he'd give it up.

But he didn't.

He came racing toward me in the middle lane, probably doing more than eighty miles per hour. I was speeding toward Tillary Street, the last intersection you cross before getting onto the Brooklyn Bridge, when two good things happened: first, the light was green. Second, there is often a police car just sitting there on the far side of the intersection, and that police car was there.

I brought my speed down to nearly a stop in the middle of Tillary Street and watched in my mirrors to see what Madman would do. If he came after me, I would have pulled over to the cop for help. But he didn't. Presumably, he saw the police car himself and that was enough for him. He made an illegal turn off of Boerum onto Tillary and was gone. In a perfect world, the cop would have gone after him and given him a ticket for the turn, but instead he just sat there. But I'm not complaining. His presence alone saved the day.

I continued onto the Brooklyn Bridge and into the haven of Manhattan, my heartbeat eventually coming down to normal as the adrenaline wore off. My passengers, who up to this point had sat there frozen in horrified silence, returned to life and started chattering among themselves about the recent movies they'd seen, not bothering to make any comment to me about our adventure nor giving pause to reflect upon how narrow the tightrope is upon which we walk through the days of our lives.

I dropped them off at 23rd and 8th.

So the second rule of road rage, avoidance of, is to keep that middle finger snug and cozy between Index and Ring. And the third rule is never, never, *never* get out of your car in anger. It's one thing if two pissed off people are making obscene gestures at each other within the safety of their own vehicles. But when one or both of them step out onto the street, the next level has been reached and that is just a curse word or two away from physical violence.

I had an incident once in Rockefeller Center in which I stopped for a man on crutches who was hailing me from the sidewalk. I had to stop beside several parked cars in order to give him accessibility and this caused a slowdown of the cars behind me. The driver of one of these cars decided to blast his horn loudly and yell something out his window as he went by, thus setting off a knee-jerk, or perhaps I should say a finger-jerk, reaction on my part. In a few moments I was confronted by a wide-eyed maniac and a drooling-from-the-mouth younger man, whom I assumed to be the maniac's son, threatening me at my side window, followed by a woman, whom I assumed to be the maniac's wife, screaming at them to get back in their car – a scene from the theater of the absurd. After satisfying themselves by calling me a wimp because I wouldn't get out of the cab and slug it out with them, they returned to their own car and drove off.

But what if I had gotten out? A likely scenario would have included pushing, punching, arrests, lawsuits and jail time. There was a tragedy in November, 2007 in which a taxi driver did get out of his cab in a road rage situation and was literally run over and killed by the other driver, a civilian. So the third rule is that it's better to be a live wimp than a dead tough guy. *Never get out of your car in anger.*

Although road rage incidents with civilians are more likely to spill out of control than incidents with professionals, nevertheless road rage between professional drivers is a far more frequent occurrence, and the great majority of these incidents involve other cabbies. And that is because driving a taxi in New York City is a sport.

That's right – it's a sport!

> Definition: 'sport: an individual or group competitive activity involving physical exertion or skill, governed by rules, and sometimes engaged in professionally.'
> *(Macmillan Dictionary for Students)*

Let me tell you something – if you ever dreamed of being a NASCAR driver but for whatever reason this occupation was not in the cards for you, the next best thing is to drive a taxi during the night shift in New York City. It's not *like* car racing. It *is* car racing.

During the day, there's too much traffic to make competitive driving a real possibility. The streets are so crowded with cars and pedestrians that you can't pick up much speed. But at night, particularly after midnight, both the number of vehicles and the number of people on the streets drop sharply. Passengers become much harder to find and it's not unheard of for a cabbie to go up to an hour without a ride. So the competition to be the first to get to whoever may be standing a bit down the road looking for your services is ferocious. And it's this competition that leads to road rage between cabbies.

Now picture this: there are sixteen avenues that pretty much extend the length of the thirteen-mile-long island called Manhattan. Most of these avenues run in one direction with synchronized lights that imitate the motion of a wave. So if a cabbie can ride the front of the wave, like a surfboarder, he will have the best chance of being the first to get to that rare and cherished passenger. The game therefore is to maintain your position on the front of the wave and not to let any other driver pass you. This means timing the speed of your taxi so you go through the light at the nano-second it turns green. Doing it safely, I might add, is quite a skill.

If there is only one empty cab going up the avenue, then that cabbie 'owns' the avenue. There is no competition. If there are two cabs, then normally one cabbie takes the left side and the other takes the right. It's when there are three or more empty cabs that things can get nasty. The one or ones in the middle will try to stay even with the other two as they ride the wave and hope that there's a double-parked vehicle or other obstruction somewhere up the road. If so, then there will be a chance to leapfrog past the cab that gets blocked out by whatever's in the way and take over his position.

There are really only three rules in this sport. They're unwritten but they're generally understood. And the rules are:

1. You don't cut in front of another cabbie in an attempt to get to a passenger before he does if cutting in front of him means that he must hit his brakes to avoid crashing into you,

2. You don't try to get to a passenger by going through a red light or making an illegal turn, and

3. You don't cut in front of a cab that's waiting in a line.

When any of these three rules are violated, then, as in other sports, it's considered cheating and there may be retaliation. Cursing at the offending driver or flipping him the bird are not uncommon. But it can get much worse.

Retaliation by the toss of an unwanted object at the cheater is one option. I have seen half-eaten fruit, bottles, lit cigarettes, chewing gum, saliva and even eggs go flying through the air at taxi drivers who didn't play by the rules. I myself have thrown apple cores and water through the opened windows of a few drivers who had stolen fares from me.

But as foolish as it is to throw something at someone, it's not nearly as foolish as using your cab as a retaliatory weapon. Here's an example: Taxi A and Taxi B are cruising along an avenue late at night, one on the left, one on the right, riding the wave. Taxi A gets a little bit behind on the wave, maybe a quarter of a block. Suddenly, a bit further down the road, the silhouette of a person can be seen standing just off the curb with hand in the air, doing the taxi hail. Taxi B, seeing that Taxi A has fallen just a little back, speeds up, cuts across the avenue, and gets to the passenger first as Taxi A screeches to a halt just behind him. The passenger, as they usually do, gets into whichever cab got to him first, which in this case is Taxi B. As the two cabs start moving again down the avenue, Taxi A retaliates by speeding ahead of Taxi B, cutting in front of him, and then braking hard, daring Taxi B to crash into him. He does this one or two more times before turning off the avenue and going his own way, feeling both disgust at having lost a fare that should have been his and satisfaction at having evened the score by intimidating both the driver of Taxi B and, most likely, his passenger as well.

These incidents are almost always brief and, although scary, rarely result in an accident. It's basically one driver telling the other, 'You can't do that to me, you miserable stupid stinking cheating bastard idiot *fuckhead*, without paying a price for it!' It's usually over in less than half a minute and, with over 13,000 taxis on the streets and over 40,000 licensed drivers, you figure you'll probably never see the jerk again and, even if you did, you wouldn't remember each other anyway.

However, this is not always the case.

Zorba

There was a period of time in 1985 when there was a driver on the streets who, due to numerous run-ins with him, became my personal nemesis. Superman had Lex Luther, Batman had the Joker, Sherlock Holmes had Professor Moriarty, and I had this guy. I dubbed him 'Zorba the Greek' because his name, which I'd seen on his hack license a couple of times, was long, convoluted and Greek and I couldn't remember it. So 'Zorba the Greek' he became.

Zorba was a guy who would stand out in a crowd. He was somewhere in his thirties with a bushy black mustache, bushy black eyebrows and a completely shaved head. How tall he was, how heavy he was around the middle, and whether or not he had one, two or six legs I could not say because, although I had seen him on numerous occasions, I never saw him from the waist down. I had only seen him from the shoulders up, sitting behind the wheel of his Chevy Caprice, driving at an outrageous speed, cutting boldly in front of me, and grabbing passengers away from me who, by any standard of fair play and human decency, were clearly meant to be *all mine.*

Maybe it was the fact that he was so recognizable that made me remember him. Or maybe it was because for that certain period of time in 1985 it seemed that whenever a fare was being stolen from me, I'd find that Zorba was the culprit. Like the time I was waiting at a red light on 7th Avenue at 14th Street and spotted a person hailing me from the other side of the intersection. It was a situation in which I would have to wait for my light to turn green, make a left onto 14th, and stop to let the new passenger into my cab. Zorba, it turned out, was on 7th Avenue on the next block, between 14th and 13th (7th Avenue runs one-way downtown). As if having eyes in the back of his head, he somehow spotted the passenger hailing me and, before the light could turn green, he backed up into the intersection and into the oncoming traffic of 14th Street, made a left, and snatched the passenger away from me.

When you're a cab driver you remember incredibly cutthroat moves like that and when you discover that the maniac doing it to you is a repeat offender, obsessive thoughts of revenge begin tap dancing in your mind, like a Fred Astaire windup doll gone mad.

Revenge! Yes, revenge…

But how?

I put my brain to work on the problem and eventually came up with an idea which seemed appropriate. 'The next time you mess with me, Zorba,' I thought, 'the next time – there will be a price to pay.'

I could hardly wait.

It took three months, but finally on a June night at eleven-thirty, there it was. I was cruising down 2nd Avenue in the far right lane, riding the wave at a speed of about thirty-five miles per hour, and as I crossed 41st Street I spotted a potential passenger on the far right corner of 40th. He stood a few feet out from the curb, waving his arm at the approaching cars – a completely normal hailing situation. According to the unwritten taxi driver code of conduct, the cab driving straight in the far right lane gets him, and that was me. I even flashed my high beams on and off at him, a communication that means, 'I see you hailing me and I will stop for you.'

And then it happened.

I was driving just a little too fast and this caused me to get ahead of the synchronization of the lights on 2nd Avenue and therefore to catch a red light, ever so briefly, at 40th Street. I stopped momentarily to wait for the light to turn green, and that moment was all that it took.

A streak of yellow came charging across 2nd Avenue from the far left lane, went right through the red light I had stopped for, and came screeching to a halt in front of the passenger, cutting me off viciously in the process. I tried to get the attention of the passenger by sounding my horn and waving my arms, a desperate attempt to beg him not to get into the cab of an animal who would cut somebody off like that, but it was to no avail. The passenger got into the other driver's cab.

I was furious. I stepped hard on the gas and pulled up so I could get a look at him. I thought to myself that in all of New York City there could be only one cabbie with enough balls and outright greed to have pulled off that move.

Sure enough, it was Zorba.

So the day of reckoning had arrived. Like a pilot of a fighter plane, I prepared for battle. First, I switched on my 'off-duty' light. Roger. Then I checked the traffic ahead on 2nd Avenue. Roger, it looked clear. Then I faded back one car length, let Zorba get ahead of me, and pulled up behind him. The key to my plan was to follow him until he hit a red light. Only then would I be able to strike.

It wasn't surprising that trying to keep up with Zorba was no easy task. As we headed down 2nd Avenue he zigged, he swerved, he zagged, and he generally drove like the madman I knew him to be. But I was not to be denied. I was determined to stay right behind him like a shadow, even if doing so was difficult and dangerous. After all, this was the day I'd been waiting for! Battle cries that must have been long dormant in my DNA began to surface to my consciousness: i-eeee, i-eeee, Zorba! Now you must die!

He went straight down 2nd Avenue for what seemed like forever, finally making a right on 9th Street and coming to a stop at a red at the next intersection, 3rd Avenue. That was good, but in order for me to execute my plan I needed to be able to come up next to him on the right side of his cab and unfortunately I was boxed out by another car in that position. Damn!

The light turned green. Zorba went straight and caught another red at 4th Avenue, but it was only a momentary red which turned green as soon as we approached it. He continued straight on 9th Street toward Broadway, the next intersection, and as we moved forward I made a bold move of passing the car in front of me which had previously boxed me out. This put me right behind Zorba, a favorable position. The light at Broadway also turned green almost as soon as we got to it and Zorba continued toward the next intersection, University Place, where a red light awaited us. As he came to a stop at University, I rolled up next to him on his right side. At last I was exactly where I needed to be.

I kept coming up beside him until my driver's side window was directly adjacent to the passenger's window in the rear of his cab. I drew his passenger's attention by tapping lightly on my horn and then motioned to him to roll down his window as I rolled down mine. The moment of truth was at hand.

'Listen,' I said, very hush-hush but just loud enough for Zorba to overhear what I was saying, 'I know this driver. His meter is way fast. Just thought you should know.'

Of course, I had no idea if his meter was fast or not, but that didn't matter. Zorba's passenger bought it in its entirety, nodding his head to show his complete comprehension and saying 'thanks' back to me in such a way as to communicate that he understood that both he and I were soldiers in the struggle for honesty and ethical business practice in the taxi industry.

Zorba's reaction was far more expressive, however. He went completely berserk.

'YOU FUGGING SON OVA BISH!' he screamed as he turned around violently in his seat, his eyes bulging in rage. If he'd been a cartoon there would have been smoke fuming out of his ears.

My bomb having found its target, I shifted into Phase Two of my strategy which was to take immediate evasive action with minimal damage to my own vehicle and person. The light turned green on University exactly on cue and I made a quick right. Watching in my mirror, I saw that Zorba was beginning to make a right as well, no doubt with some kind of retaliation in mind. However, his passenger didn't want him to make a right – he wanted to go straight. Zorba's cab came to a stop for a few moments in the middle of the intersection, then swung back again on 9th Street in the direction of 5th Avenue. As I watched them disappear from sight, the passenger was sitting forward in his seat in a rage of his own, giving Zorba a chewing out that he so richly deserved.

I can't say for sure what the full effect of my vengeance was on Zorba. Maybe he crashed into a wall and died. Maybe he was strangled by his passenger. Or maybe this was the last straw for him and he decided to get himself into a line of work more fitting to his own personality, like stealing pocketbooks from old ladies or becoming a 'repo man' (the guy who takes your car away when you fall behind on your payments). Because I never saw him again.

Years went by without any more serious road rage incidents for me. Of course, there were occasional flare-ups with other cabbies and a few garbage truck drivers, but things were relatively peaceful. It appeared I had mastered control over my own impulses.

Yeah, right…

The cure

I have to confess that what sets me off more than any other stimulus is when another driver appears to me to be nothing more than a sadistic bully who thinks he can use his car as his way of pushing other people around. Evening the score with someone like this takes on the significance of not just putting this one particular bully in his place, but of putting all bullies who ever lived in their place and eradicating bullydom for all future generations. It becomes a *cause.*

I was cruising down 2nd Avenue in the left lane at around 7 a.m. one night in April, 1989, when I was hailed by a middle-aged woman who was standing on the curb at 62nd Street. Seeing her waving at me, I did what I am supposed to do in this situation: I pulled over as close to the curb as possible and stopped. She then did what she's supposed to do in this situation: she opened the left rear door of my cab and began to get in. That's pretty mundane, isn't it?

Well, it was unacceptable to the driver of the car that was directly behind me. Like the driver who harassed me near the entrance to the Brooklyn Bridge, this guy decided his inconvenience was too much to bear in silence and showed his displeasure by sounding his horn repeatedly. I, however, having perhaps mellowed with experience, did not respond. There was no middle finger coming out of my window nor any other retaliation. I just ignored the guy.

My passenger got in and, after agreeing with me that the guy blowing his horn must be a complete idiot, told me she wanted to go to Queens. In those days there was an entrance onto the Upper Level of the 59th Street Bridge right there at 62nd Street, so I made a left and then a quick right onto the ramp. Just after I made that turn I saw in my rearview mirror that the horn blower was speeding up and was about to pass me. That's the expected reaction from a motorist who sees himself as having been victimized by another driver. The psychology here is that he has been made 'effect' and now, by passing the person who stopped him, he is putting himself back at 'cause'. It was no big deal to me. I see it all day long.

But what happened next I do not see all day long: the driver, a guy maybe forty years old, and his girlfriend sitting next to him, were both giving me the finger as they passed me on the ramp! And they were laughing with each other in a mean sort of way. It got to me.

'I'm not gonna take that,' I said to my passenger.

'Damned right,' she replied, 'you show them.'

Her comment was unexpected and quite welcome. It's not every day that you have a cheerleader backing you up as you head into a road rage incident. I made a quick decision as to what I would do and went ahead with it. I sped up to about sixty miles per hour and passed *him*. When I was a car length ahead I moved in front of him and then did something I knew would drive him completely insane:

I slowed down gradually to about ten miles per hour.

Now, his reaction to this was, of course, to try to pass me again.

But when he pulled out I pulled over, too, to prevent him from passing. He then pulled over the other way and I did the same. We zigged and zagged several times and I could see in my mirror that the guy was completely livid. My passenger was loving it and kept cheering me on and the thought crossed my mind that she might be one of those women you see in the audience of a boxing match with an ecstatic look in her eyes as she watches two men punch each other into Happyland. After half a minute of this, realizing that just possibly it was going too far, I let him go by.

Not unexpectedly, he then cut back in front of me and drove even slower than I was driving. But by this time the incident was over in my mind and I refused to retaliate. He seemed to have had enough of it, too, and picked up his speed, putting some distance between us and making the light at the end of the ramp. I did not make the light and when it turned green I made a left onto the street there, Thomson Avenue, only to find a big surprise waiting for me.

Several 'brownies' – the slang name given to the Traffic Department personnel in brown uniforms who direct vehicles – were standing in the middle of the road, pointing at me and ordering me to pull over. After I did so and stepped out of my cab, I was confronted by the angry, horn-blowing, middle-finger-waving bully who had just tangled with me on the bridge, and he was holding something up near my face that I found most disturbing: a police badge!

Oh, damn, the guy was a cop.

'Give me your driver's license and your hack license,' he ordered with a scowl.

I started to say something in response, but he cut me off and repeated the command. He then added, almost shouting,

'I'm gonna get you for reckless endangerment, I'm gonna get you for dangerous lane changing, and you can forget about being a cab driver. I'm gonna get your hack license, too.'

I went back into the cab and retrieved the documents, along with my trip sheet and a pen. After handing the two licenses over to him, I told him I wanted to see his driver's license, too, since he did the same thing to me on the bridge that I did to him, and I had a witness.

He glared at me and held up his badge again.

'This is all the identification you need,' he growled. I wrote the number down on my trip sheet as he began to copy my information into a notebook.

Meanwhile, my passenger had gotten out of the cab and was squaring off verbally with the cop's female companion, who turned out to be a cop, too. The whole thing was beginning to look like some kind of a bizarre tag team match, man against man and woman against woman. The brownies stood off to the side, seemingly amused by the spectacle.

With visions of a huge fine and a revoked hack license dancing through my head, I thought it would be wise to try to cool things down, if possible.

'Listen,' I said to the cop in a civil tone, 'why were you making obscene gestures at me when you passed me on the bridge?'

He stopped copying down the information from the licenses and paused, looking at me from over the top of his notebook. After a few seconds he replied in a surprisingly civil tone of his own:

'I wasn't making obscene gestures at *you*,' he said, 'I was making obscene gestures at *her*,' indicating my passenger. *'She gave me the finger when she got in your cab!'*

Uh, *what?*

And with that revelation he finished writing down the information, got back in his car with his colleague, and drove off. It was one of the few times in my life I would describe myself as being truly dumbfounded. I just stood there and watched them drive away.

My passenger, however, got back in the cab in a state of exhilaration. Apparently her head-to-head with the female cop had released some pent-up energy and had done her some good. She gladly offered to come forward as my witness if I needed her and gave me her contact information. That was really nice of her, and was greatly appreciated, but it turned out to be unnecessary.

I never heard from the cop again.

So there is this fourth rule you must always remember when it comes to avoiding road rage incidents. And that rule is:

Everyone is a cop!

That mean-looking moron who cut you off and you're about to flip the bird to? He's a cop. That guy in a Prius who's going too slow in the passing lane? A cop. That stupid kid on a skateboard? Isn't that something, they're letting children on the police force now. An old lady with a cane? Definitely a cop, what a clever disguise.

They're all cops! Remember this, and I promise you'll be cured forever of the urge to partake in this activity.

They're all cops!

11

Karma versus Coincidence

Was it karma? Or coincidence? That is the question.

New York is a city of particles in motion. People everywhere, all kinds of people – moving; cars, buses, bicycles, motorcycles, trucks – moving; and of course taxicabs, thousands of taxicabs – moving, moving, *moving!* The assumption is that all these particles have no higher intelligence controlling them and that when they happen to bump into each other it's just a coincidence.

But what about this?

One night in 1987 I picked up a blind woman who asked me at the end of the ride if I would accompany her into the lobby of an apartment building so I could ring the buzzer of the person whom she was about to visit. Being that she was blind she could not, of course, read the names above the buzzers. I was happy to do this and the incident of being able to help her in such a unique way was gratifying to me and remained in my mind. I'd already been driving a cab for ten years at that point and this was something that had never happened before. In fact, it was something I'd never even imagined happening.

Then the next night *another* blind woman got in my cab and asked me to do the same thing! Again I accompanied a blind passenger into the lobby of an apartment building and rang the buzzer for her. And it has never happened again since.

Karma or coincidence?

Or how about this?

I was cruising in Midtown one evening in the summer of 1985 when a middle-aged man got in my cab who wanted to go to LaGuardia Airport. He was friendly and talkative and, since I had a baseball game on the radio, the conversation soon turned to baseball. He lived in Miami, he told me, but had grown up in Los Angeles and had always been a Dodger fan. Suddenly, and quite unexpectedly, he handed me a baseball card – *his* baseball card; that is, a baseball card of himself. On the front it showed a color picture of him in a Dodger uniform holding a bat on his shoulder. On the back there was a brief biography: 'Silver Bullet [his nickname], a left-handed line drive hitting forty-six-year-old rookie, had two game-winning hits and was a defensive standout leading Albuquerque to the 1985 championship at Dodgertown. Look for him on the parent club in spring.' He told me the card was mine to keep.

Although it was quite genuine-looking, my passenger was not a professional baseball player. He had attended a 'fantasy camp' earlier in the year, something that many Major League teams offer, for a price, to fans who want to spend a week in Florida in the off-season playing baseball with some of the former players from their favorite team. One of the extras you can get at these camps is a baseball card printed up of yourself, also for a price.

We spent the rest of the ride talking about his experiences at the fantasy camp, which he spoke of with such enthusiasm that it made me think it must have been one of the highlights of his life. When we got to LaGuardia, as an acknowledgment to his fantasy, I asked him to autograph his card for me, which he gladly did. He then left the cab with a big smile and a wave goodbye and when I got home I stored the card inside one of the notebooks I used to use to record my taxi-driving experiences.

Six years later, in the summer of 1991, I was again cruising in Midtown, looking for a fare, when I picked up a middle-aged man en route to Gramercy Park. Since I had a baseball game on the radio, the conversation again turned to baseball. My passenger then told me he was a Brooklyn Dodger fan as a kid (the Dodgers played in Brooklyn before moving to Los Angeles in 1958) and that his father used to own a clothing store that hired Willie Mays, the star player of the hated Giants, as a pitchman. Suddenly, completely out of nowhere, he handed me a baseball card of himself wearing a Dodger uniform, with a glove on his left hand as if he was about to catch a ball. It was almost a duplicate of the one I'd been given years earlier, with a color photo on the front and a brief biography on the back: 'Dion [his nickname] enjoys baseball, football, and hockey. His goal in life is to play 2nd base for the LA Dodgers and to be a rock and roll star in the '50s and '60s'.

He, too, had attended a fantasy camp hosted by the Dodgers. He, too, spoke about the experience with the greatest of enthusiasm. I wondered if he was the same man I'd had in my cab in '85, and I told him I thought he might have ridden with me years earlier and given me his card then, but he replied that was impossible because he'd only been to the fantasy camp once, and that had been earlier that year, 1991, and it had been a Christmas present from his wife. We spent the rest of the ride talking about the fantasy camp and what a great time he'd had and he left the taxi with a big smile. This card, too, was mine to keep.

I contemplated what the odds were here. I had never met anyone in my life before 1985 who'd ever shown me a baseball card of himself. I didn't even know these things existed. So what were the odds that I would ever get not one, but two of these cards randomly given to me in my lifetime? And to take it a step further, what were the odds that both of these cards would be from the same team?

When I got home that night I dug out the first guy's card. He was indeed a different person. But wait, his first name was Larry. The second guy's first name was also Larry. What are the odds that, added to the other unlikelihoods that already existed, the only two people I've ever met who had baseball cards of themselves would also have the same first name? A million to one?

But there was more. The first guy's last name was Silver, and the second guy's last name was almost the same, Silver*man.*

Twilight Zone music, please. And then that question – karma or coincidence?

Now you could make an argument that both this and the incident with the blind ladies were coincidences. Highly unlikely coincidences, but coincidences nevertheless. Okay, I could give you that. Coincidences do happen, after all.

In fact, one of the favorite games of regular taxi riders in New York is called 'I Think I've Been In Your Cab Before'. The conditions of this game are: over 13,000 taxicabs, over 40,000 licensed drivers, and about one million rides a day. It would be an interesting exercise for an actuary to figure out what the odds are of getting the same driver twice. It does happen, and many passengers keep track of these things, as do I. Here are some of my favorites:

- One evening I picked up a man and dropped him off at his doctor's office on Park Avenue. Later that night I picked him up again, this time coming from the hospital where his doctor had sent him for tests, and took him back to his apartment building.

- I picked up a young man and a young woman at 25th and 2nd. A moment after they got in the cab the guy says, 'I think I was in your taxi a few days ago.' He recalled the conversation we'd had, about how certain streets got their names, and I remembered the ride myself. Turning to the young woman, he said, 'This is the cab driver I was telling you about.' Well, this was quite flattering and we continued on to their destination, a restaurant in the Village, in great spirits. After dropping them off, I drove around the city picking up and discharging passengers for the next two hours. Then I picked them up again coming out of the restaurant where I'd left them and we returned to 25th and 2nd.
- In the early '90s my driving schedule was the night shift on Sundays, Mondays and Tuesdays. One Tuesday at about 5 a.m. I picked up a young man on the Upper West Side and drove him to Penn Station. The following Sunday I was waiting in the taxi line at Penn Station and this same young man, accompanied by his wife, appeared and got in my cab. It turned out he and his wife were actors who were performing in the road company of *Phantom of the Opera* which at the time was playing in Philadelphia. When I'd dropped him off at Penn Station he'd been on his way to Philly to begin the week's schedule with a Tuesday night show. When I picked them up on Sunday night they had completed the week's performances and were coming home to their place in Brooklyn for their two days off. So this young man was taken to the train station and picked up from the train station by the same driver – me.

Okay, I am admitting that all these incidents could be nothing more than coincidences. But what about *this?*

Special delivery

In 1980 I decided to write a full-length stage play and dedicated myself for the next year to completing it, which I did. Then, having this manuscript in hand, I was trying to figure out what to do with it. One idea was to contact a documentary filmmaker, a New Yorker, whom I didn't know personally but was a friend of a friend. His name was Bert Salzman and he'd won an Academy Award a couple of years earlier for one of his movies, a documentary. So, even though my stage play was not directly in the area of his art, I thought he could potentially lead me in the right direction if I could get him to read it. So I obtained his home address from my friend and sent him a letter introducing myself, asking if he'd be willing to receive the manuscript.

Several weeks went by and I had not received a reply. Then one night I was cruising up 1st Avenue in the Upper East Side and a man and a woman got in my cab headed for the Upper West Side. The gentleman looked familiar. I looked at him carefully in my mirror. Was it possible? My God, it was Bert Salzman!

'Bert Salzman?' I asked, already knowing it was him.

Although he had received a good measure of fame by winning an Academy Award, documentary filmmakers do not expect to be recognized by their cab drivers. He was a bit startled.

'Yes,' he replied cautiously.

'Did you get my letter? I haven't heard back from you.'

I believe the thud I then heard was Mr Salzman's jaw dropping to the floorboard. The result was that he very kindly did read the manuscript and offered me some helpful advice.

Now, if you think *that* was a coincidence, then this is where we part ways. Although we may not know the science of it, surely something is going on here. After years of observation of this phenomenon, it is my opinion that one of the key ingredients in this thing we call 'karma' is the factor of attention. It would seem that when one's attention is either stuck on or is causatively put on a particular thing, there is some kind of mechanism put into play that sends that thing your way.

Not a laughing matter

At 10.31 p.m. in 1990 I was cruising in the Theater District on West 45th Street, looking for my next fare. It's a time when the theaters are letting out and it should have been easy to find a passenger. In fact, I would have bet money that before I'd reached 8th Avenue I would have had a paying customer in the back seat, yet for some reason that was not happening. As I approached the end of the block, I drove by the Music Box Theater and noticed that a crowd of people had gathered around the stage door. The drama *A Few Good Men* was playing there (it was produced on Broadway before becoming a movie) and, as is common after a show, a crowd of theatergoers were showering a departing performer with affection. Through the corner of my eye I noticed that the person exchanging pleasantries with the crowd was an actor, Tom Hulce, who had starred in one of my all-time favorite movies, *Amadeus.* In that movie he played the role of Mozart and had imbued his character with a particularly idiosyncratic, high-pitched laughter that wonderfully communicated the unsophisticated raw talent of the genius composer. It was a performance I very much enjoyed.

Immediately the thought occurred to me that it would have been really cool if Tom Hulce had gotten into my cab. As I drove up 8th Avenue hoping to find another passenger, I started imagining what I would have said to him. That laugh was certainly the thing I would have wanted to hear and I wondered how I might have been able to get him to do it. I came up with an idea - I would have let him know that I knew who he was, I would have told him how much I liked *Amadeus*, and then, as a joke, I would have offered him a ten percent discount on the ride if he'd give me that laugh from the movie. I thought this would have been hysterical and wondered where the brilliance came from that enabled me to envision such hilarity. I must be a genius myself, kind of like Mozart, but pushing around a yellow box instead of pushing around *Symphony No. 40* and *The Marriage of Figaro* and all that other stuff.

I cruised up 8th Avenue and finally found a passenger at 55th Street. After I dropped him off on the Upper East Side my fantasy about getting Tom Hulce to laugh crept back into my universe. The concept was so funny to me that it was staying with me as a form of mental self-amusement. But after another ten minutes it began to fade and my attention returned to the more mundane activities of a typical shift in the life of a taxi driver. I took two more fares around town, one to Tribeca and the other one returning me into the vicinity of Times Square. It was 11.30 p.m.

I drifted around Times Square and before long I found myself once again crossing 45th Street between Broadway and 8th Avenue looking for that elusive fare. By now, though, the street was almost empty. The shows were all over and the theatergoers had cleared out, so I didn't expect to find a passenger right there on that street. I started thinking about what route I should use to increase my chances of finding my next customer, but as I neared the end of the block the door of a bar opened and a solitary figure emerged with that 'I want a taxi' look on his face. I pulled over and stopped before he even had a chance to lift his hand in the air.

And Tom Hulce got in my cab.

'23rd and Broadway, please,' he said.

There was a surreal moment here – to the effect of, 'is this really happening?' – but I quickly recovered and sprang into action. After establishing our route, downtown via 9th Avenue, I turned on the chit-chat button. A little weather, a little traffic, and then, say, you look familiar to me, are you an actor? Tom Hulce? Oh, Tom Hulce! I saw you in *Amadeus*, I love that movie! Are you doing something on Broadway? *A Few Good Men*? Oh, I heard it's great, what's it about?

Tom Hulce turned out to be quite friendly and a ready conversationalist. I asked him a bunch of questions about *A Few Good Men* – its plot, the other actors, the reviews, who wrote it, how long it would probably be running on Broadway, and so on, and he told me all about the show. I found his comments interesting, but, of course, my interest in it was just a ploy. My ulterior motive was to keep the conversation going until I felt sufficient rapport had been established to enable me to move in for the kill. And when we got to 23rd and 7th I made my move.

'Say, you remember that laugh you did in *Amadeus*?' I asked.

'Sure,' he replied, rather flatly.

'Boy, do I have an offer for you! If you would do that laugh for me right here in the cab, I'll give you a ten percent discount on the ride! How's that for a deal?'

'It's sweet of you to ask,' he replied, 'but I'll have to say "no".'

'You *won't?*'

'Sorry.'

I was startled and disappointed. Here I was, all set to be entertained and I was coming away without even a giggle.

'All right,' I countered, 'make it fifteen percent!'

This brought a smile, but no laugh. Seeing that there was no wiggle room here, I had no choice but to come to grips with the fact that the Mozart laugh was simply not on the market, apparently at any price.

But it didn't get me down. After dropping him off at 23rd and Broadway, I found that I was happy enough to be glimpsing beyond the door of the physical universe and into the realm of metaphysics. I am of the opinion that human beings are spirits inhabiting bodies – actually trapped in bodies – and are inherently capable of things like extrasensory perception and out of body perception. And I think the concept of karma is more understandable if one takes the point of view that thought itself is senior to the world of matter, energy, space and time.

Still, you may be skeptical. Okay, then, how about *this*…

The actress

It's possible that my own personal karma in regard to thespians and the theater in general may be quite volatile, because, aside from Tom Hulce not laughing in 1990, there had been a prior karmic squall with an actress nine years earlier. For two weeks in 1981 she kept showing up like a psychic boomerang. That wouldn't have been a particularly negative experience had she been a pleasant or even mildly annoying individual. But she was one of the most obnoxious pains in the ass that ever walked the streets of New York and the fact that she kept appearing out of nowhere could only lead you to wonder what the hell was going on here.

It all began with my friend Harry, with whom I was sharing a rented taxi in those days. We would alternate use of the cab – Harry would take it for three days, then I would drive it the next three days, and so on. It was a workable arrangement in that we both made money and we both had time off. On the turnover day, Harry and I would get together and discuss, among other things, any interesting incidents or passengers we'd had in our cab during the previous three days. It was at one of these conferences that I first became aware of 'the actress'.

Harry was usually a pretty upbeat guy, but on this particular day, as we met over breakfast, I could see he was a notch down from 'upbeat'. I asked if something was bothering him.

'I can't get this woman who was in my cab last night out of my mind,' he said. 'She drove me *crazy*!'

Harry went on to explain that he was driving in the Theater District looking for a fare at around the time the shows let out when a woman came rushing through the crowd, shoved her way past two other people who were approaching his cab, and jumped in. Calling the people 'idiots' whom she'd just barreled over, she ordered Harry to drive her to 87th and York Avenue, and to drive quickly if he was really a cab driver and not just another jerk pussyfooting around in a yellow car. She went on to explain, without having been asked to explain, that she was starring in a Broadway play called *Gemini* and that she made more money in a month than most people make in a year.

Harry said he decided to humor her for the sake of keeping the peace and to just acknowledge whatever she said until he could get rid of her, but it wasn't easy. She was, he said, the worst back seat driver he'd ever encountered. She told him which route to take to get to 87th and York, which lanes to drive in, when to speed up, and when it was okay to stop. She even told him to run red lights, but Harry had his limits when it came to running red lights. He would only run them if he'd checked first to make sure there were no cops around, a habit which she found rather annoying.

'Why didn't you just throw her out?' I asked.

'Well,' Harry said, 'she was a character. Besides, for some reason I thought she'd be a good tipper.'

'What'd she give you, a dime?'

'Twenty cents on a $3.80 fare. Exactly 5.26 percent.' Harry was always good at numbers.

'And the part that really got to me,' Harry continued, 'was that she decided to tell me that the reason my tip was so small was because I told her I didn't remember seeing the commercial for her show on TV. She said they've been running the same commercial for years and everybody's seen it and that I must be full of crap if I'm telling her that I haven't seen it.'

'*Have* you seen it?' I asked.

'I didn't think so at the time,' Harry said, 'but now I think I might have. She said it's the one where a woman hits an actor who's supposed to be her son and tells him to "take human bites". She's the woman.'

'Oh, yeah,' I said, 'I've seen it.'

'Well, maybe you would have gotten a better tip than I did,' Harry said.

I sympathized with my friend. The fare sounded like a horror story and I could see why it would still have been on his mind the next morning. Our conversation finally turned to other matters and I had no further thought about the actress. Little did I know that a karmic wheel had been tipped off its pedestal and was going to come rolling over me.

It arrived at 6.30 p.m. that very same day. I happened to be cruising for a fare on the Upper East Side, at 86th and York, when I was hailed by a doorman. I pulled over and a middle-aged blonde entered my cab.

'Get me down to 45th and Broadway,' she barked, 'and get me there fast.'

'Oh God,' I thought, 'what a bitch.'

'Take 86th over to 2nd, get in the left lane,' she snapped. 'That jackass in front of us is going too slow, get around him.'

'Lady,' I replied, 'are you bleeding from a gunshot wound or something? What's the big rush?'

'I'm the star of a Broadway play. I have to get to the theater. I said to get *around* that guy, come on!'

'Really? Which play?'

'*Gemini* – have you seen the commercials on TV?'

'Are you the one who says, "take human bites"?'

'Yes, that's me!'

'I don't believe it! I share this cab with my friend, Harry. You were in his cab last night. Harry was your cab driver. He told me about you.'

'Is that right? What did he think of me?'

'Well,' I said, suddenly realizing I was heading for thin ice here, 'he said you were… a *character*.'

'Well, tell your friend Harry that I'm more than a *character*. I'm a star and I make more money in a week than he makes in a year.'

'Oh.'

'Now make a right on 79th. Don't stay in this lane. Go down to 5th. You can make that light, step on it, come *on!*'

Harry is not a guy who is always right, but he was as right as right could be on this one. She was an undiluted maniac and she rode me like an evil jockey the whole way down to the Theater District. By the time we got down there I felt like I'd been worked over by a couple of thugs.

'You ought to come see the show sometime,' she said as she prepared to leave the cab. I was a little dizzy by this time and not really thinking about what I was saying as I blurted out,

'I don't really get to the theater much anymore.' I guess that wasn't tactful enough.

'Well,' she shot back, 'I guess we'll just have to survive without you.' And with that she handed me some money and walked off in a huff.

The fare was $3.70. She'd given me four dollar bills – a thirty-cent tip. Harry was right again. I'd told her that I'd seen her commercial and I *did* get a better tip than he'd gotten. Beat him by a dime.

I drove the remainder of that night in a particularly less cheerful mood than when I'd begun it, and when I woke up the next morning I was still brooding internally about the slap down I'd received from the actress. I probably should have called Harry right away to get the thing off my chest, but I waited until we met again on turnover day and laid it on him over breakfast at the T-bone Diner in Forest Hills. Harry was duly amazed.

'Where would you put her on your all-time list of worst passengers?' he asked me.

I thought about it for only a moment.

'Definitely in the top five,' I replied. Harry nodded knowingly. We ordered our eggs and continued squeezing the topic of conversation for any further significance we could find in it. One of the things we touched on was the idea that if the three of us (me, Harry and the actress) were, in fact, caught up in some sort of karmic tug of war, what would it take to break the cycle?

Funny we should have mentioned that.

Harry drove the cab for the next three days. At the beginning of the fourth day – turnover day – we again met over breakfast. When I laid eyes on Harry, I could see he was on fire.

'Wait 'til you hear *this*!' he all but shrieked.

'Don't tell me you had her in your cab *again*!'

'I *did*!'

Harry told me the story before the first cup of coffee had arrived. He had picked her up the previous night at 86th and York, as I had, and once again the Theater District had been her destination.

'I can't believe it!' Harry had said to the actress. 'This is the second time in a week you've been in my cab and, not only that, you were in my friend's cab a few days ago. He told me all about how he'd had this whole conversation with you, and all.'

'Really,' the actress said, 'what did he think of me?'

Harry was ready for her.

'He said you were one of the five worst fares he's ever had,' he answered matter-of-factly.

If this had been a movie, it would have been the part where the bad guy takes a bullet, grabs his chest, and falls down dead in a cloud of dust on a lonely street in the center of town. The cautious heads of the townsfolk would slowly start appearing from behind windows and doors and the hero's sweetheart would come running up and kiss him passionately, tears of joy streaming down her cheeks. The sun would set, the sound of righteous music would fill the theater, and 'THE END' would appear on the screen.

Instead it was a taxicab in Manhattan and there aren't any lonely streets and the townsfolk barely notice things like bad guys taking bullets. Nevertheless, the desired effect had been achieved. The actress slumped back in her seat and said not another word for the duration of the ride.

Call it an exorcism if you want. Call it purification by fire or call it a stake through the heart. Call it what you will, it did the trick – whatever Force brought the actress to us was ready to whisk her away again. And the proof of this took place later that night when she appeared before me *again.*

I was cruising up 8th Avenue looking for a fare at 10.30 p.m., just the time when the Broadway shows are letting out. As I approached 44th Street I found myself immersed in a sea of automobiles due to the fact that hundreds of people all trying to find a cab at the same time creates a traffic jam. And then there she was, coming right at me in the center of 8th Avenue.

The actress didn't stand near the curb and hail a cab like the rest of the human race. She marched right out into the middle of the avenue amidst the moving cars and stalked out her prey. But

I saw her coming and, like a creature of the wild doing what it must to survive, I followed my instincts and reacted instantly.

Using the automatic switch, I locked all the doors and at the same time flicked on my 'off-duty' light. Nevertheless the actress approached me with her arms waving frantically and tried in vain to open the right rear door. She then pounded it with her hand, but it was no use. I ignored her and kept moving, not unlocking the doors until I could see in my rear-view mirror that she was seeking out a new cab driver to victimize in the middle of 8th Avenue and I was out of harm's way.

And that was the last I ever saw of her. *Gemini* soon closed and apparently took the actress with it, perhaps into someone else's karma problems. And the streets of New York, I want you to know, have been safe ever since.

Mean old hags

Well, maybe not completely safe. There was one particularly nasty squall of karma which occurred not too long after the actress had been swept off into another universe. It featured the mean old hags.

I was driving a Friday night shift and it was one of those nights when business seemed to be everywhere. That's the way you want it to be if you're a cab driver – one gets out and the next one gets in in rapid succession. Do that for a few hours and you've made yourself some *mucho dinero.*

At about 7.30 p.m. I pulled over to the curb on 79th Street between Park and Madison to drop off a passenger. As I was being paid the fare, a rather pathetic sight appeared a few yards in front of me on the sidewalk. It was an elderly man attempting to walk to my cab who was supported by not one, but two crutches under his arms. He managed to lift one crutch into the air to hail me and, as I was accepting money from the passenger who was about to leave, I signaled to him with a wave of my hand that I had seen him and that the cab would be his.

But no sooner had my departing passenger opened the rear door to leave than the door on the other side of the cab was suddenly opened by a well-dressed, white-haired woman who moved with the speed of a gazelle in planting her butt on the back seat and thus claiming the cab for herself. She was joined in the blink of an eye by a second white-haired woman and I was informed, before I could utter a syllable, that their destination was 91st and Madison. It put me in an awkward position.

'Actually, I was already hailed by that man on the sidewalk with the crutches,' I said.

'Well, that's just too bad for him,' the first woman snapped back, 'let's go.'

I had a split second to decide what to do. I found myself confused and hesitant, and then I took the coward's way out. I made a facial expression to the man on crutches as if to say 'sorry' and then pulled the taxi out onto 79th Street and started to drive off. But the thing wasn't sitting well with me and I felt a need to let these pushy women know what I thought.

'Well,' I said sarcastically, 'I guess that just shows the kind of civilization we're living in.'

The second woman was right there on the uptake.

'If we want your opinion, we'll ask for it,' she barked.

Ouch.

I brought the cab to a stop at a red light at the end of the block, where 79th meets Madison, and the temporary break in the ride gave me the time I needed to collect my thoughts and decide what was the right thing to do. I added up the pros and cons of the situation and came to the conclusion that if decency, justice and fuzzy little kittens were to have any place in the future of this planet, there could be only one correct way to proceed: these mean old hags had to *go.*

Now, I have a confession to make. I used to have a device in my cab, quite illegal, which was an easy solution to the problem of what to do with unwanted passengers. It was a secret cut-off switch. Flick the switch and the engine would die. When the ignition key was then turned to try to start it up again, the engine would turn over but it wouldn't catch. A few curse words regarding that 'damned fuel pump', an apology to the passengers, and bingo, they were *outta there.* It was painless and no one was the wiser.

So when the light turned green, I made a right onto Madison and, before I reached the intersection at 80th Street, I turned on the cut-off switch and right on cue the engine sputtered and died. I went through my script about the fuel pump and even went out onto the street and opened up the hood of the cab, just to create the right effect. To my delight, they bought it in its entirety, paid me what was on the meter, and in a moment they were standing out on Madison Avenue looking for another cab.

I was hoping I could rub it in by closing the hood, starting the engine, and driving off without them, but unfortunately they somehow found an available cab almost immediately. But no matter. Justice had been served. I was greatly satisfied and, I must admit, rather smug about the way I'd been able to so adroitly dump them. I made a left on 81st Street and headed toward 5th Avenue in search of my next fare. It was going to be a good night after all.

As I made the left onto 5th I was hailed by the doorman of a building that is one of those places that's so exclusive that in order to live there you not only have to be a millionaire, you have to be a well-connected millionaire. Two white-haired ladies got into the cab and I had the thought as they sat down that, God, you know they look just as mean as the two I'd just gotten rid of.

'Take us to 151 East 75th Street,' one of them demanded.

'Yes, ma'am,' I said, trying to sound pleasant and sincere. I pulled out into the traffic on 5th Avenue and headed downtown. 151 East 75th Street was going to be between 3rd and Lexington Avenues and, due to the one-way directions of most streets in

Manhattan, this meant I would have to drive past 75th Street to 74th, go east to 3rd Avenue, and then make a left on 75th in order to get them to their destination. It was garden variety navigation. I do this twenty times in a shift.

I wasn't paying too much attention to my new passengers as I drove down 5th. They were talking quietly to each other and my thoughts had returned to my victory over the forces of evil back on Madison Avenue. I drove past 75th Street and pulled into the left lane to prepare for my left turn onto 74th.

And then I heard it.

'*You passed the street, dummy,*' the voice said, just loud enough for me to take notice of it.

'WHAT DID YOU SAY?' I shot back incredulously, as I glared at them in the rear-view mirror.

'I said you passed the street,' the woman sitting directly behind me said with a snarl, leaving out the 'dummy' part. She was just a little, white-haired lady but I swear I saw fangs jutting out of her mouth. I pulled the cab over to the curb and stopped.

I turned around in my seat and confronted them.

'Did you say, "You passed the street, *DUMMY*"?' I growled with venom in my voice. Now *I* was the one who had fangs.

'Well, if you had half a brain you wouldn't have passed the street,' she replied.

Now you've got to understand something here. With all the thousands and thousands of passengers I've had in my cab after driving for all these years, I'd never, *never* had anybody talk to me like this. It just doesn't happen. And now I had two sets of them in a row, a double dose of mean old hags. Coincidence? Forget about it, it was karma in a most undiluted form, and an instinct that I didn't fully understand at the moment suddenly guided me in knowing just what I needed to do to free myself of its grip.

'GET OUT!' I screamed at the mean old hags. This was no time to be sneaky and use the cut-off switch. This was the time to look the tiger straight in the eye.

They just sat there and said not a word.

'GET OUT OF MY CAB!'

They still weren't getting the message. I opened my door, walked to the rear of the cab, opened their door, and repeated the command. I was quite willing to physically remove them from the premises, and I was about to do so, when they finally realized they were dealing with a madman and got out on their own volition. We exchanged mutual curses under our breaths and went our separate ways.

And that was the end of mean old hags, once and for all. Since that time whenever a white-haired lady has gotten into my cab she's been sweet, somebody's grandmother, and from Indiana or somewhere.

For the trick to being at cause over one's karma, I learned, is being able to confront its source in its entirety. For what can be fully viewed will vanish, which is to say that it will no longer have an effect on you. And that's the truth of the matter.

12

The Animals of Manhattan

Manhattan is a man-made universe. Although it's an island and at ground level it's basically a slab of rock, it's hard to imagine that only a few hundred years ago it was a wilderness with trees and streams and Indians running around on dirt trails. One might think that all those coffee shops, newsstands and potholes had been here forever.

Along with the flattening of the land and the removal of any obstruction that got in the way of Man, the animals that used to call this place home were also shown the door. If you travel a mere twenty or thirty miles from Midtown, you will still find plenty of animals living in their natural habitat as they've been doing for countless centuries. But not in Manhattan, Charlie. It's humans only, so take a hike.

Unless you're a pigeon. Pigeons are allowed and, in fact, do quite well here (just try running one over. It can't be done). Sparrows, chipmunks, squirrels and mice are also thriving. And, of course, the rats. It's been said there are more rats than humans in New York City, but I think that number includes the owners of taxi garages, so perhaps it's an exaggeration. In any case, there are plenty of them around.

Even most insects have a difficult time making a go of it in Manhattan. There are hardly any bees, wasps or mosquitoes. Beetles are rare. Ladybugs, scarce. There aren't too many ants around. Flies, however, are doing all right, as are the bedbugs. And cockroaches – well, what can you say? Cockroaches are the exception to the rule and are doing so well that I once drove a shift from hell in a cab that was infested with them, a night I will never forget. You get the idea that if they can make a taxicab their home, they can adapt to any environment and probably will indeed still be here long after we humans are gone. My hat's off to these creatures, especially when I'm making sure they're not in there, too.

Given these few exceptions, Manhattan is a place where you'd better be a human or at least a pet of one. Right?

Stranger in a strange land

On the night of February 28, 2010, as I was cruising down Columbus Avenue on the Upper West Side at around 2 a.m., I had to brake to avoid hitting a pedestrian who was crossing against the light at 79th Street. Well, actually, I probably wouldn't have hit the pedestrian since he turned out to be a One Inch Wonder – he had timed his movement so that he would just barely make it across the avenue before being run over. This, of course, isn't unusual in Manhattan where we have so many daredevil jaywalkers. What *was* unusual was that the pedestrian wasn't a human – he was a coyote!

Realizing I was witnessing an extraordinary event, I brought my cab to a halt as the five or six other vehicles on the avenue proceeded downtown without me. The coyote paused on the sidewalk at 79th and for about ten seconds, separated by not more than thirty feet, he took a good look at me and I took a good look at him. I had thought that perhaps it was a dog, but as he turned to face me I could see that, although they were quite similar, this was no Fido. He had a wolfish face and an independence in his bearing that was not like that of a domesticated animal. It was definitely a coyote.

My immediate thought was to get his picture. I carry a camera with me at all times that sits beside me on the front seat and I grabbed it. But, as often happens in street photography, by the time I had the power on and had brought the viewfinder up to my eye, my subject had moved away, trotting into a four-block-long park that surrounds the back of the American Museum of Natural History. He was gone.

Nevertheless, I knew I might still have a great photo opportunity on my hands, so I pulled the cab over to the curb, took camera in hand, and walked into the park at 79th Street in pursuit. The coyote had gone north, toward the park's 81st Street boundary, and I caught sight of him again from a distance of about one block. There then began a fascinating game of cat and mouse (so to speak) between the two of us.

Envision this scene, if you will: just myself and this animal in a snow-covered park at two in the morning, with no pedestrians on the streets and the only sounds to be heard coming from the occasional rumblings of automobiles moving down Columbus Avenue. The stillness, silence, cold air and light from a full moon imitated the ambiance of the wilderness, so very unlike Manhattan, while a mind game was beginning to take place between a human and an animal. The coyote had caught sight of me and was aware that I was following him. Whenever I moved, he moved. When I stopped, he stopped. And, as if to frustrate me, whenever I was about to snap his picture, he would move again.

I spent about ten minutes trying to get a decent shot until he finally exited near 81st Street, went back out onto Columbus Avenue, and lost me. After I returned to the cab and checked how my pictures had come out (not so great), I had a few reflections about the experience. First, how completely odd and curious it was that, of all the locations he could have wandered into, he chose the grounds of the Museum of Natural History. It was as if he was consciously seeking sanctuary in the one place that humans have set aside for the study and understanding of nature and its creatures.

Next, how incredible it was that a shift of taxi driving could be interrupted by a wildlife adventure in the middle of Manhattan. That is surreal.

And finally, I found myself empathizing with the plight of the poor coyote. He had somehow wandered away from his natural habitat and found himself a stranger in a very strange land, a feeling I've often had in my own life.

A couple of days later, the presence of at least two coyotes on the Upper West Side was reported in the media. About a week after that, one of them was finally cornered by the police in Chelsea, tranquilized with a dart, and eventually released up in Westchester County, north of Manhattan. It was speculated that the coyotes had come into the city via train tracks that run alongside the Hudson River. The other one, I'm happy to say, was never found and it's assumed he returned from wherever he'd come. Unless perhaps he somehow got into the Museum of Natural History and has been posing there as a stuffed animal ever since!

So, given the rarity of wildlife suddenly showing up on Columbus Avenue, what we are left with, as far as animals in Manhattan are concerned, are pets. And in Manhattan, there are two kinds of pets: indoor and outdoor.

Indoor pets could be anything, from gerbils to tigers (yes, in 2003 there was a much-publicized story of a man who kept a four hundred pound tiger in a room in his apartment in a Harlem housing project). The trouble with indoor pets, though, is that we don't generally ever get to see them. Indoor pets are a private affair. Outdoor pets, on the other hand, are a public affair and are monopolized by the one animal that is as much a part of New

York culture as the bagel and the metro card. I speak, of course, about our beloved dogs.

It's odd, if you think about it, that in a humans-only world there should be this one particular animal that is so commonly accepted as a member of the club. By my own estimate, I believe there are close to a million dogs in the city. If you'd never been to New York, you might think this would be a problem, but it's not. Dogs are usually very well cared for, and there is no such thing as a stray anywhere. This is a statement I can make as someone who drives around the city all night long. I *never* see a stray dog. Stray cats, yes, and stray humans, certainly, but never dogs.

Another thing I never see (well, almost never) are canine souvenirs on the streets of the city. This was not, however, always the case. Way back when, dodging doo was a part of every New Yorker's day. But the pooper-scooper law (the living legacy of Mayor Koch) in the '70s made not cleaning up after Rover a social faux pas. Today, every New Yorker walking a dog knows that the eyes of the citizenry are upon him. Fail to bathe for a month, wear shoes that don't match, beat your wife, walk around with a Bush/Cheney button on your jacket – hey, all right, these things can happen. But fail to clean up after your dog... *you just try it, mister!*

So it is inevitable, with their huge population in the city, that a taxi driver will from time to time be asked by a passenger if it would be all right if a dog comes along for the ride. You notice I used the word 'asked' – this is because cabbies are not required by the rules to take animals in their cabs unless they are service animals, like seeing-eye dogs, or in cages. When someone is transporting a cat, for example, it is almost always in a carrying-case. And the one time I had an animal in my cab that was neither a dog nor a cat, it was also in a unique transporting device. It was a parrot. A woman who worked in a big Midtown law firm was traveling with her pet bird, the 'office parrot'. She said it brightened up the workplace both for the attorneys and the clients without being too obtrusive. She carried it in a special container which had glass windows so it could be seen during the ride. The beautiful green and yellow parrot brightened up my taxicab, too.

As years have gone by, I have had hundreds of dogs in my cab, including one celebrity dog, a black Lab, which was coming from the *David Letterman Show* after stuffing some amazing number of tennis balls in its mouth for the 'Stupid Pet Tricks' segment. I've never refused to take a dog since I like them and their presence in my cab is a guarantee of a pleasant conversation with its owner. Many drivers, however, will refuse to let dogs into their taxis. Some say this is due to fear of the animals or to a clash with cultural values in which it is considered beneath the dignity of a man to give service to a dog. I, however, think I know the real reason. It's because here is an opportunity to pass somebody by *legally!* There are so many times a cabbie drives right past someone for whom he is required by law to stop and then suddenly here's this chance to do it without having to worry about getting a summons. There must be a certain irresistible attraction to that.

The truth is, it is less risky to take a dog in your cab than it is to take a human. I've never had a dog who was drunk. I've never had a dog throw up in the back seat. I've never had a dog beat me for a fare. In fact, I've never had any problems with dogs at all.

Well, perhaps that is not a completely truthful statement…

Rambo

Rambo was not a muscular lunatic with a machine gun. He was a Doberman pinscher who was traveling with his owner, a friendly, twenty-something guy whose name I didn't get. They jumped in at 75th and 3rd one night in August, 1987, and were en route to Alphabet City via 2nd Avenue. I was introduced to Rambo and told what a loyal, cuddly and generally wonderful companion he was.

'It's great having a big dog in this city,' my passenger said. 'I take him with me whenever I can. If someone raised a hand to me, Rambo'd probably tear the guy's arm off. So I always feel safe when he's around.'

That was a discomforting comment but since it didn't apply to me I didn't think twice about it. We zipped down 2nd Avenue having a lively conversation and making all the lights. When we got to 11th Street he pointed to a deli and asked me to pull over so he could go in and buy a couple of things while I waited for him. Not a problem.

I stopped the cab at the curb and he jumped out with a 'be right back' as he closed the door behind him. It took me two or three seconds to realize that a) Rambo wasn't with him, b) uh-oh, Rambo was still in the cab with me, c) the cab we were in had no partition in it to keep us apart, and d) up to this point, contrary to his reputation, Rambo had not been a particularly friendly dog. He hadn't been unfriendly, but he wasn't one of those abundantly affectionate ones, either.

But not to worry. All I had to do was show him that I was a nice guy and meant him no harm. I turned around in the front seat so he could see my winning smile.

Big mistake. Rambo barked at me, loudly, and then gave me that scary mad dog snarl with his teeth showing.

I froze in fear, literally unable to move. Rambo barked again, then started to pace back and forth with great agitation on the rear seat. He looked out the window toward the deli and barked again. Then he sat down and began staring at me while the sound of a frightening low growl started coming in my direction through the spaces between his teeth. I got the feeling that if I made even the slightest motion, he'd jump forward and make a hamburger out of my neck. Remember, Dobermans are the ferocious-looking dogs you see in World War II movies that are always on the side of the Nazis.

My life kind of flashed before me. Especially the part when my mother tried to talk me out of driving a cab because of how dangerous it is. A city full of criminals, murderers and weirdos – none of whom had ever given me any trouble – and now I'm going to get killed by a dog.

We sat there, Rambo and I, in frozen confrontation for what seemed like an hour in death-by-dog time but was probably more like sixty seconds in waiting-for-passenger-to-return time. Suddenly our showdown was interrupted by a loud noise on the street – a driver on 2nd Avenue was sitting on his horn and yelling at another driver. It startled Rambo. He turned to his right and barked at the source of the commotion.

It was my opportunity. I turned around and grabbed my door handle, opened the door, jumped out of the cab, and slammed the door behind me in Olympic-record time. Rambo was left in the cab by himself.

It took me about a minute to catch my breath and by then my passenger had emerged from the deli, a small bag of groceries in hand. He was all smiles. I wasn't, and told him about my struggle for survival with his dog. Apologizing profusely, he explained that Rambo hadn't eaten all day and 'he gets irritable when he's hungry'. He pulled out a can of Alpo from his bag and held it up for me to see.

'That's why I stopped at the deli. Sorry.'

Well, no harm had been done – I checked and found that I still had all my fingers - so we got back in the cab and I dropped them off at Avenue A. Looking back, I'd say it was the scariest thing that's ever happened in my cab, if you don't count the time I had a drunk inspector from the Taxi and Limousine Commission riding with me as a passenger who kept showing me his badge, turning the meter on and off, and urging me to go with him into a certain bar.

But that's another story.

Unconditional love

The American Aristocracy on Park and 5th Avenues has its millionaires, its billionaires, its debutantes, its Very Important People, and its Very Important Dogs. You get to rub noses with them all if you're a cabbie.

Most of these passengers are pretty boring, but two of them made quite an impression on me one evening in January, 1981. They jumped in at 64th and Park, dressed in bright, plaid outfits. Both had cute, wavy hair and both had the manicured nails of the smart set. Those were the dogs. Their owner, a tinted blonde of about fifty, wasn't dressed quite as fashionably, but she didn't look too bad, either.

It was a straight run up Park to 92nd Street. I felt I had to make a comment about the dogs – they were begging for attention.

'What kind of dogs are they?' I asked, as they nestled in her lap.

'Yorkies,' she replied.

'Ah, Yorkshire terriers,' I said, 'those are a couple of beauties.'

She beamed with pride.

'Yes, they are my wittle puppie-wuppie Yorkie-Warkies,' she said, and she puckered her lips and made kissing gestures at them without actually touching them.

She pointed at the dog on her left and made an introduction. 'This is the precious Isabelita,' she said, and, pointing to the other one, 'this is the precious Bartholomew.' Then she spoke directly to the dogs. 'This is the cab driver, buppies.' Apparently I was neither precious nor did I have a name. But no matter, I couldn't be offended. I played it straight.

'How old are they?'

'Just four months,' she replied. Then, leaning forward and lowering her voice to a whisper, she said, 'They're going to get their S-H-O-T-S.' Each letter was pronounced distinctly to allow me time to spell the word.

'Oh!' I said, a bit too loudly. 'You're going to see the vet!'

She whispered again.

'Yes, to the D-O-C-T-O-R.'

'Would they be upset if they knew where they were going?'

'Why, of *course*!' she asserted, and she kissed at them again as if to reassure them of her enduring love in case they happened to have overheard where their destination was.

We stopped at a light. I turned around and reached over to give the little dears a pat on their heads. As my hand approached them, she pulled them back.

'Please, they just had their hair done.'

Well, stupid me.

'Oh, sorry,' I said. The light turned green and we drove on, getting closer now to our destination. 'Have you considered entering them in shows?' I asked.

'Absolutely not!' she shot back. 'The pressure on them would be dreadful!' I tried to imagine what form this pressure could take and all I could think of was the dogs bursting out into tears as they found out they had not been chosen 'best dogs in show', and then needing years of therapy to undo the damage. How sharp and cruel are the daggers of life.

We had arrived at 92nd so I made a right and stopped in front of a building between Park and Lex. She paid the fare, added an average tip to it, and, before leaving, asked me to come out and open the door for her, which I did. She stepped out of the cab with a dog tucked snugly under each arm, thanked me, and entered the building where I assumed there must have been a veterinarian.

I suppose there are things I could say about this lady regarding how tightly or not tightly her head was screwed on. I could say she thought more of canines than she did of humans. There might be a lot of things I could say, but there's one thing I couldn't take away from her: as far as those dogs were concerned, she had the makings of a fine (shhh, I'm going to whisper this now)... M-O-T-H-E-R.

Now, Isabelita and Bartholomew are able representatives of the type of pet we most often see on the streets of New York, but the indoor pets do occasionally make cameo appearances, too. Like a boa constrictor wrapped around a woman's neck in Central Park. Or a parrot on someone's shoulder. Or a ferret on a leash. Or the guy who was often seen walking around Times Square late at night with a cat balanced *on his head*! (I've got the picture to prove it.)

And then there are the circus animals. Each year when the Ringling Brothers, Barnum and Bailey Circus comes to town they do a publicity stunt of walking the camels, zebras and elephants through the Midtown Tunnel at around one in the morning. I once sat in traffic on 34th Street watching them hoof it westward toward Madison Square Garden and I remember thinking the experience would have been complete if only I'd had the foresight to bring along some Cracker Jacks.

Exotic animals which have no business showing up in Manhattan are sure to grab your attention, but there was one in particular who'd been around so long that I eventually barely even noticed him.

Whatever you say, buddy

For a couple of years in the early ’80s on any given night in the warm months you could predictably find, either in front of the Hilton Hotel on 6th Avenue or a few blocks up the street on Central Park South, a man and his llama.

The man had, as you might expect, a Peruvian look to him, wearing a serape over his shoulders and a wide-rimmed hat on his head. The llama was white, saddle-bagged, bridled, and had that permanent llama smile on his face that I’ve always found charming whenever I’ve seen one in the zoo. There was a placard attached to the animal espousing some cause, but whether it was animal rights, Peruvian rights or some other kind of rights I never knew because I never bothered to slow down enough to read it. But what I did know was that I had seen the two of them so often that eventually this incredible sight of a llama in the middle of Manhattan seemed just a part of the scenery to me and, as mentioned, I hardly took notice of it.

One hot July night I picked up a drunk yuppie on 45th Street and 6th Avenue at around eleven o’clock. He wanted to go to 3rd Avenue and 70th Street, so we headed straight up 6th. The guy was a talking drunk, the kind who just talks and talks without much caring whom he is talking to or whether or not anyone is really listening to him. The best way to handle such a person is the 'uh-huh' approach. Whatever he says, you just say 'uh-huh' back. There's no point in trying to get into a real conversation with him because he's not really there, he's just sloshed. So you 'uh-huh' him for ten minutes until he's out of your cab.

The guy was laying it on thick about his girlfriend.

'She wants to get married and have a baby,' he said, 'so she can quit her job.'

'Uh-huh.'

'I'm not marrying anyone 'til I have a quarter-mil in the bank. If that takes me another two years, she'll just have to wait.'

'Uh-huh.'

'I just have my priorities, you know what I mean?'

'Uh-huh.'

'I'm not saying I don't want to marry her. She's great. We've been living together for six months now and I don't screw around on her, either.'

'Uh-huh.'

'I just have my priorities, you know what I mean?'

'Uh-huh.'

We were approaching Central Park South, where 6th Avenue ends. I made the right turn and headed east toward 5th. Standing there, in front of the St Moritz Hotel, was the man and the llama. I barely noticed them.

My drunk yuppie lunged to his right and pointed out the window.

'Holy shit! Did you see that?' he screamed.

'What?' I asked casually.

'There's a fucking llama over there on the sidewalk!'

'Uh-huh,' I said.

He turned around and looked through the rear window as we

moved across Central Park South.

'Oh my God! There's really a llama back there! Did you *see* that?'

'Uh-huh. A llama,' I said flatly.

He reached forward and placed his hand lightly on my shoulder.

'Listen, I'm not kidding,' he said, almost pleading with me, 'there's really a llama over there, okay?'

'Hey, buddy, if you say there's a llama, then there's a llama.'

'I'm not *saying* there's a llama, there really *is* a llama!'

'Okay,' I said, 'there's a llama. Right there on Central Park South.'

We moved quickly across 5th Avenue, then continued through Madison, Park and Lexington, catching all the lights. I made a left onto 3rd, caught a red at 60th Street, and then started moving uptown again. All the while Mister Yuppie was trying desperately to convince me that he'd really seen a llama and all the way I was doing nothing but agreeing with him.

Finally we pulled into the driveway of his high-rise on 70th. A doorman came out to open the door as I was being paid the fare.

'Johnnie, you're never going to believe what I just saw over on Central Park South – a llama!'

Like cab drivers, doormen know how to humor drunks.

'Is that a fact?' the doorman said, with just the slightest trace of skepticism.

My passenger sensed that he was being patronized.

'You don't believe it? Just ask *him*,' he said, pointing at me. Johnnie looked at me and made a facial expression asking if this could be true. I motioned to him to step over to the cab so I could say something out of earshot of the passenger, and he came over.

'You know on Central Park South where they've got all those horse-drawn carriages?' I asked.

He nodded.

'Well, apparently one of them is a llama tonight,' I said, and I did a little pantomime of bringing a glass to my lips, as if to say, 'This guy's had one too many.'

Johnnie smiled knowingly and walked back over to the guy. As I pulled out of the driveway I glanced in my rear-view mirror for one last look at the two of them, and I could see that my passenger was starting all over again to try to get Johnnie to believe him that, hey, man, really, *really*, I'm telling you, there really was a llama back there. On Central Park South. A llama! Really!

I know it was a cruel thing to do, but I just couldn't help myself. The poor guy is quite possibly still trying to convince people to this day that he once saw a llama on Central Park South.

But who would believe that?

Everybody knows that Manhattan is for humans only.

13

In a Rush

An athletic-looking young man throws himself in the back seat and blurts out, 'Penn Station – as fast as you can!'

A redhead tells me she's going to Soho, then adds, 'and I'm late!'

A middle-aged businessman employs tact when saying that he doesn't want me to do anything illegal, 'but if you could get me to Charles and West 4th in ten minutes, you would be saving my life'.

And a grumpy old frump fails to employ tact as she barks, 'Make the light!'

As a connoisseur of the subject, I speak with some authority when I tell you that there are two types of 'In a Rush':

a) passenger is late, and

b) passenger is in crisis mode.

The great majority of rush rides are the former, passenger is late. It's a straightforward affair – we start at Point A and the passenger is supposed to be at Point B by a certain time. We can either make it or we can't. The crisis mode rides are much more adventurous, of course. A cabbie may very suddenly find himself in a life or death situation that requires great speed. Although what's a matter of great urgency to one may not be cause for alarm to another.

One evening, for example, a woman got in at 82nd and Madison. With great stress in her voice she told me she needed to get to 64th and 1st absolutely as quickly as was humanly possible.

'Please, please,' she begged, 'do whatever you can. I don't care if you have to run red lights, please just get me there!'

I happen to be touchy on the subject of running red lights since that has proven to be a rather expensive habit in the past, but if it was really a matter of life or death, I would consider putting my license at risk. I asked her what the big rush was all about. It turned out there was a pet store at 64th and 1st and she needed to get to it before it closed so she could purchase nail clippers and a certain shampoo. Her friends were coming over to her place that night and Reggie, her Boston terrier, had to look and smell his very best.

Unkempt dog = major crisis.

At eleven o'clock that same night I was hailed at Broadway and 106th by a man who put another man into my cab who had a towel wrapped around one of his fingers. The first man gave me $10, telling me to get the other man to Emergency at St Luke's Hospital as quickly as possible. As I pulled away, I asked my new passenger what was up and he said that he worked in a restaurant and had just sliced one of his fingers 'most of the way' off. I told him to hang on and that I'd get him to the hospital in a flash.

'No, don't sweat it, man, just drive like you always do,' was his response.

Holding your finger together with a towel = no big deal.

*

So a cab driver has to get smart at discerning what's worthy of driving at seventy miles per hour for and what's not. If you've been stung by a few pretenders, you may start to become unresponsive to passengers' pleas for haste. But a cabbie should not forget that there are also certain instances where there can be no doubt that you've suddenly found yourself in the middle of a true crisis.

Dinner with Doctor K

I was driving up 1st Avenue one evening in September, 1989, at 7.30 p.m. when I spotted a middle-aged gentleman in a tuxedo hailing me on the east side of 52nd Street. Tuxedo equals big event so I expected to be directed to drive to Lincoln Center, a major hotel or a fancy restaurant, but his destination turned out to be an apartment building on Washington Square Park in Greenwich Village. I thought that meant we'd be picking someone up and then continuing on to wherever the big event would be, but that wasn't it, either.

'I want you to wait for me while I go upstairs, then take me back to where you picked me up,' he exclaimed with just a trace of a smile on his face. 'And if this thing's got wings, make it fly! This is an emergency!'

I immediately figured out what the fastest route would be at that time of the day, then bolted across 1st Avenue with a little screech of my tires, just to show him I was on board. I made a left on 53rd and went over to 2nd Avenue, which would be our downtown route to the Village. I knew there must be some kind of a story attached to this ride and I kind of suspected from his smile that he wanted to tell me about it, so I asked him what his big emergency was all about.

He told me he was the president of NYU (New York University, the largest college in New York City) and that he'd just arrived for dinner at the residence of Henry Kissinger, only to find out when he got there that it *wasn't* formal, meaning that he was about to be the only man at the dinner party dressed in a tux! So what we had to do was race back to his apartment so he could change into a regular suit, then race back to Dr K's. Dinner would be served at eight.

It was a social disaster in the making which had to be averted by any means. I told him I could get him there in twelve minutes and back in twelve minutes, so he'd have six minutes to go upstairs and change his clothes. In actuality, I got him there in eleven and back in ten, running a couple of red lights along the way. Amazingly, it took him only five to change into a suit, which may have set a new *Guinness Book* record and gotten him thinking about switching his occupation into that of a quick-change artist. We arrived back at 52nd Street with four minutes to spare.

Plenty of time to grab an aperitif and an hors d'oeuvre or two before being seated. *Bon appetit, monsieur le president!*

Now, when dealing with passengers in crisis mode, you might think that the phrase 'follow that cab!' would pop up with some frequency. It certainly does in the movies. But in all my years of driving, I have heard it used for real only twice (but lots of times as a joke). Once when a passenger realized he'd just left his brief-case in the back seat of another cab and used my cab to catch up to it. And another time when a man wanted to follow his lover and her husband a few blocks just to see where they were going.

What you don't see in the movies as often but which does happen every once in a while is the opposite of 'follow that cab' – '*lose* that cab'. A woman once jumped in at 5th Avenue and 84th Street and, after driving a few blocks, told me we were being followed by someone in another taxi, a person with whom she didn't want to have any contact. She asked me to see if I could give it the slip, so I did a little action scene of zigs, zags, and quick turns resulting in a successful evasion. Another time I picked up a 'shemale' coming out of a tranny bar late at night in Midtown and after getting on the West Side Highway and driving a couple of miles, she told me we were being followed. I didn't believe it at first, but it turned out to be true. A U-turn, some speed, and running a red light left the stalker in the dust.

Occurring a bit more frequently than 'follow that cab' or 'lose that cab', however, is 'beat that cab'. This happens when the situation arises of there being too many people to ride in a single taxi, so they split their group up into two taxis which are both going to the same destination. Some wise guy in one cab thinks it would be fun to race the other cab and challenges the driver to get to Point B first. I've had many such races and I'll tell you something – it *is* fun.

The race for the nipple

Starting line: West 4th Street and 6th Avenue in Greenwich Village.

Personnel: Four twenty-somethings in my cab – a guy sitting next to me on the front seat, two girls and another guy in the back. Three of their friends in a second cab just to my left.

Finish line: 36th Street and 3rd Avenue in Murray Hill, a distance of about two miles.

It was a Saturday night at 2 a.m., so, not surprisingly, they were all somewhat sloshed. The fellow sitting up front with me felt an inner need to entertain his friends at my expense, so he went at it.

'Hey,' he blurted out so everyone could hear him, 'we've gotta beat them there!' I gave him a shrug of my shoulders and a look on my face as if to say that I didn't have much interest in racing with another cab.

He noticed.

'Come on, man, I know you're the man! I know you can beat that other cabbie! I *know* you can do it!' His friends in the back were all for it, chiming in with grunts of encouragement.

I sensed a business opportunity opening up.

'Oh, yeah?' I asked with a smile, 'so what's in it for me?'

He thought about it for a moment and then made a grand pronouncement:

'You will be kissed by those two beautiful girls in the back seat!' he proclaimed. The girls just sat there smiling. It was a nice offer, but it didn't motivate me. I wanted something more tangible, something I could take to the bank.

'How about some *money?*' I suggested. 'Give me a dollar amount.' Kisses I didn't need. Dollars I did.

The guy turned out to be a shrewd negotiator. Not wanting to part with more money than he had to, he counter-offered.

'Okay,' he said, 'here's the deal. If we get to 36th Street first, my girlfriend will show you her nipple.'

I looked again in the mirror. Both girls were still smiling. I looked at the guy. He looked at me.

'Deal!' I exclaimed. Here was something worth racing for. Yes! I wanted that nipple!

And we were off.

The light turned green and I headed uptown on 6th Avenue. My first order of business was to figure out my route. No problem, it was obvious – straight up to 23rd Street, right turn, straight across to 3rd Avenue with the great flow of green lights that 23rd has if you're traveling eastbound, then a left on 3rd and up to 36th. I was hoping the other driver would choose another route, but he must have been an experienced cabbie because he went the same way I did. It was definitely the best way to go.

Sixth Avenue, like all the one-way avenues in Manhattan, has the lights synchronized in a 'wave', so this other cab and my own were traveling beside each other all the way up to 23rd Street, not stopping even once as each light turned green as we approached it. My passengers, particularly the guys, became my cheering section.

When we finally did catch a red at 23rd Street and 5th Avenue, we had a short break in the action. The guy in the back seat got on his cell phone and informed his friends in the other cab that we were in a race to see who would get to 36th Street first. This brought the excitement level up a notch as now there was not only a nipple at stake, there was professional pride.

The light turned green at 5th Avenue and the race continued. Both myself and the other cabbie knew we would get greens at Madison, Park and Lexington Avenues and then we'd have a red at 3rd. So it was a matter of jockeying for position so that one of us would be in front of the other at that 3rd Avenue red. I was in the lead the whole way, and then the moment of truth arrived: just as we approached 3rd Avenue, he tried to cut in front of me. I held my ground and sped up enough to close the small gap between my cab and the car in front of me, forcing him to pull in behind me. That was the critical move of the race.

When the light turned green at 3rd Avenue, we both made left turns and went one block toward a new red light at 24th Street. Other vehicles were already at the 'line' except for one open spot on the left which I grabbed. This meant that when the light turned green I would have no cars in front of me and I could zip all the way up 3rd Avenue. The competing cab would be stuck behind other cars.

And that's exactly what happened. I coasted up 3rd to victory at 36th Street, bringing the taxi to a halt on the far right corner of the intersection. And now it was time for my reward.

I turned to look back at the girls, wondering which one was the girlfriend who was about to be the prize-giver. But both rear doors had been quickly opened and the guy and one of the girls were already outside the cab, with the other girl moving hastily toward the exit.

I turned back around and looked at the fellow sitting on my right.

'So… where's that nipple?' I asked. A man has a right to collect what's owed him.

With what might be called a shit-eating smile on his face, he called out to his girlfriend.

'Hey, Jess…'

But Jess was already out on the street.

'I'm not *that* drunk!' she called back as she closed the door behind her.

I looked again at the guy. He shrugged his shoulders and had an expression on his face that said that he wished he could help but was powerless to do so under the circumstances.

'Some pimp you turned out to be!' I groaned in mock distress.

The fare was $8.60. He gave me $11, a bit more than the usual ten for that ride, but I was not placated.

I wanted that nipple!

God spits on me

It was a Sunday around noon on a cloudy day in October, 1982, and I was heading toward Manhattan on Queens Boulevard, hoping to get a fare into 'the city' (as Manhattan is referred to by people who live in the other four boroughs). I was hailed in the section of Queens called Sunnyside by punkish-looking guy, about twenty years old, wearing the uniform of the alienated youth – a black leather jacket, some chains, and an earring or two. He jumped in and told me he wanted to go to the East Village – 3rd Street and Avenue A – and he wanted to take the Brooklyn–Queens Expressway to the Williamsburg Bridge, one of three bridges that connect Brooklyn to Manhattan.

I was delighted. It's like money found when you get one of these rides. Manhattan is where you were going anyway, but now you're being paid for it. So I made a left on 43rd Street from Queens Boulevard and in a couple of minutes we were on the BQE, heading for the Williamsburg Bridge, as planned. It is, in fact, the most direct route to 3rd Street and Avenue A, so I knew the kid knew his way around town. Probably a native New Yorker.

Punk outfit notwithstanding, he turned out to be a good conversationalist. He asked me some questions about taxi driving, I asked him some questions about himself, and we were both enjoying the ride. And we continued to enjoy the ride until we exited the BQE and entered the ramp that leads onto the Williamsburg Bridge. That's when we came to a complete standstill in an enormous traffic jam.

I grimaced in agony. Damn! I'd forgotten that the inbound traffic on the Williamsburg is always trouble on Sundays. This is because the bridge leads out, on the Manhattan side, onto Delancey Street, which is overfilled with stores that are super-busy on Sundays. As a result there's a big traffic jam on Delancey which in turn ties up the bridge.

If I'd thought of this when the kid first got in my cab, I'd have insisted on going another way. But now it was too late. We were stuck, and stuck badly. It was probably going to take half an hour to get across the bridge. It was that bad.

Our conversation dwindled. After a couple of minutes and a couple of clicks on the meter, during which time we moved about twenty yards, my passenger was beginning to get the idea that this ride was going to be quite a bit more expensive than he'd originally planned. The tension was palpable.

We crawled along for a bit until the cab came to a complete stop, and then he did a very strange thing – without any notice to me, he suddenly opened his door, stepped halfway out of the cab, and surveyed the situation on the bridge. He then got back in and closed the door. It was really weird that someone would do this. What was he going to do? Walk?

'How's it look?' I asked, knowing that it had to be awful.

'Pretty bad,' he said, showing some frustration in the tone of his voice. 'Pretty bad,' he said again, more to himself than to me.

Well, of course it was bad, but there was nothing anybody could do. We were both stuck – he was losing some money and I was losing time in which I could have been making a lot more money if the cab had been in motion. But *c'est la vie*, right? I was pleasantly resigned to the situation and was hoping he would be, too, so I started to chat it up again, thinking I could divert his attention away from our traffic difficulties. But we moved just a very short distance in the next five minutes and there's only so much chatting two people can do when they're surrounded by gloom.

After inching forward for a short bit, we came to a complete halt once again, and then the kid repeated his bizarre action. He stepped halfway out of the taxi, looked around, but this time instead of getting back in, he put his other foot out and was now standing with both feet on the bridge. What was *with* this guy?

And then it came, those dreaded words. Syllable by syllable, they shot out at me like little stones from a slingshot.

'Listen,' he said, *'I'm gonna get out here.'*

And with that, he handed me a fistful of dollars.

I was stunned. I immediately remembered the lunatic who had left me stranded in the middle of the 59th Street Bridge a couple of years earlier. I didn't think this could happen to a cabbie twice in the same lifetime. I had to say something fast.

'Hey, man,' I pleaded, 'don't walk on the bridge. It's dangerous, man. What if the traffic starts moving? You'll be stuck out there with cars zipping all around you! Tell you what – I'll turn the clock off 'til we get off the bridge. That way it won't cost you so much.' This wasn't just a matter of economics. I really didn't want the kid to get himself killed.

'No, man, thanks,' he said, 'but it's not the money. I'm in a really big rush.'

And as he said this he reached into the cab and lifted an object up from the seat. It was something which he'd been carrying with him when he'd entered but which I hadn't paid any attention to at the time.

It was a skateboard.

'See ya! Sorry!' he called out as he closed the door behind him and quickly disappeared on the thing in the narrow lane between the two rows of unmoving cars.

I counted the money. He'd given me a dollar tip in addition to the fare. Not bad for a kid, but it did little to appease my misery, which had just doubled. Now I was not only sitting still in an endless traffic nightmare, I was also not getting paid a dime for it.

The people in the car next to me had noticed what had happened and were laughing about it. One of them called over.

'Looks like one of those days,' he chuckled.

I answered by making a facial expression that was meant to say, 'This is God spitting on me'.

I sat suffering on the damned bridge for another twenty minutes before finally touching land on the island of Manhattan. A black cloud seemed to settle in around me, telling me this was the lousy beginning to what was sure to be a lousy day. As miserable as I was, though, I had to hand it to that kid: *he'd come armed with a superior mode of transportation!*

Now a passenger who gets into a cab with Plan B on his lap would certainly have to be a clever person. But I would still give the blue ribbon for Smartest Passenger In A Rush to anyone in what I would call the 'Genius Category'.

The wisdom of the carrot

Let's look at it from my point of view. During the course of every single shift I'm going to get two or three or four passengers who jump in my cab and tell me that they're in a BIG rush. The implication, or direct message, being that I need to get them there fast-fast-*fast!*

Well, there's nothing wrong with that. I don't fault anyone for telling me what his situation is. But there's just one problem – it doesn't motivate me to do anything extraordinary to help them solve something that is *their* problem. I will just acknowledge what they said and drive them to their destination in the same way I would have driven if they hadn't said anything at all. But I won't run red lights, make illegal turns, or drive ten or fifteen or twenty miles per hour faster than I normally would drive.

What they have failed to do is to tell me specifically what's in it *for me.*

Now, some passengers will make the infamous statement that they will 'take care of me' or will 'make it worth my while' without getting into exactly what they mean by that. Unfortunately experience has shown conclusively that what follows this promise is an average or even a below-average tip.

Thus a seasoned cabbie translates 'I will take care of you' as

'Hey, stupid fuck-head, I want you to go ahead and risk a fine or a suspended license and in exchange you will get nothing special.' It's an insult.

But every once in a rare while – and I do mean rare – a person will get in the cab who understands that the best way to get me to solve *his* problem is to tell me why it's in my own best interest to make it *my* problem.

One night in January, 2007, a twenty-something jumped in at Grove Street and 7th Avenue South in Greenwich Village at exactly 11.51 p.m. His destination was Fulton and Gold in the Financial District, a short ride that required knowledge of lower Manhattan's geography. I pulled out onto 7th, quickly figured out the route in my mind, and told him how I intended to go. This was meant as a passing comment, not really requiring discussion, but it turned out my passenger was quite concerned about getting there as soon as possible and wondered if another route might be better. I told him the way I wanted to go was the best way (which it was), and then he said the magic words…

'My fiancée's birthday is at midnight and if you can get me there before then, I'll give you $10 over the meter.'

Bingo! *His* problem became *my* problem.

I immediately turned into a NASCAR racer, zig-zagging my way around the Holland Tunnel traffic, making the difficult and crucial green light at Canal Street, flying down West Broadway to Duane Street, catching the greens on Church and Broadway, circling around City Hall Park and somehow making the light at Ann, and finally delivering my passenger to Gold and Fulton at 11.58.

The fare was $7.80. He gave me a twenty and happily told me to keep it. But before he rushed out of the cab, I acknowledged his brilliance by sharing with him this bit of information which

I will share with you, too.

It took me eight years of taxi driving before I noticed how rare it was for someone to offer me a specific reward for doing something special for them. Once I became aware of this, I started to count the number of times it would happen and have kept this tally in my mind. That was in 1985. Since then, the number of times a passenger has offered me a specific reward for getting him to his destination on time is... (drum roll, please)... NINE!

That is correct. Nine times. Thousands and thousands of people have told me they are in a big rush and only *nine* have had the wisdom to offer me a specific reward if I could solve their dilemma for them.

I believe there's a huge life lesson to be learned here.

Let's call it the wisdom of the carrot.

14

The Traffic Jam Hall of Fame

The mortal enemy of In A Rush, its natural predator, is Traffic Jam.

A businessman from Boston who has twenty-five minutes to get from Midtown to LaGuardia to catch the last flight out is doing just fine until the traffic comes to a complete stop on the Grand Central Parkway – there's been a three-car pile-up and all lanes are closed.

A family of four with tickets to *The Lion King* gets into a cab on a Saturday night at 8th Avenue and 17th Street with twenty minutes to make the curtain at the Minskoff in the Theater District. It should be doable, but the traffic on 8th slows to a crawl at 35th Street – a city official has allowed 8th Avenue to be closed from 42nd to 56th for a street fair.

On a December evening in 1993 a Broadway hopeful leaves her apartment on the Upper East Side, grabs a cab, and heads for an audition in Times Square. She arrives forty-five minutes late and, despite humbling herself by begging, is turned away at the door. President Bill Clinton is in town and has decided to do some

Christmas shopping in Saks, bringing the evening rush hour to its knees.

Traffic jams come in two varieties: the predictable and the unpredictable. The predictable can be dealt with. You know the traffic on 2nd Avenue is going to pile up for a few blocks as you approach the 59th Street Bridge, so you factor this into the equation. It's the unpredictable that drive you insane. I mean, who expects to be hitting a stop-and-go on the Henry Hudson Parkway at two in the morning? Here is agony in the raw.

Now, most of them are caused by roadwork that you didn't know was going on until it was too late, by accidents or by civic idiocies. But there are also jams that turn out to be the result of something so weird, so completely unique, that they deserve recognition as the gourmet items that they are. They warrant a special place where they can be memorialized for all time. What they need is… the *Traffic Jam Hall of Fame.*

A pawn in their game

After dropping a passenger off in the Park Slope section of Brooklyn at 3 a.m. on October 14, 1979, I decided to call it a night. I was tired from having been out on the streets for eleven hours and there's not much business left at that time, anyway, so enough was enough. It was time to go home, which in those days was in Forest Hills, Queens.

I flipped on my off-duty light and drove down Flatbush Avenue to its very end at Tillary Street. There I made a right turn and proceeded three blocks to the entrance of the Brooklyn–Queens Expressway, the fastest route home. But the ramp was closed – a police car with flashing lights blocked the way.

No doubt there had been an accident on the BQE and a clean-up was underway. This is something not that unusual, unfortunately. The BQE is one of the worst highways in New York City with tons of trucks and reckless macho morons in their Camaros and Firebirds, so I was annoyed but not baffled. However, it meant choosing an alternate route and that was a headache. Brooklyn has a scarcity of highways and taking the local streets back to Queens would take forever. So I decided to go back to Manhattan across the Manhattan Bridge, shoot uptown on 3rd Avenue, and then take the 59th Street Bridge to Queens. It was a route that was longer in distance, but shorter in time. I turned my cab around and was on my way.

The streets in Manhattan are empty at that time of the night, so it took only five minutes to get all the way from Chinatown to Murray Hill, a distance of about two and a half miles. And then the oddest thing happened. I hit a solid wall of traffic at East 30th Street and 3rd – the entirety of the avenue was filled with cars and they weren't moving an inch, a sight you never see at that time of the night. Looking up 3rd Avenue, I noticed helicopters hovering above a building a few blocks uptown and a bit to the west, and I knew immediately what was going on.

Fidel Castro was leaving New York City.

The bearded dictator had been in the city for four days to make a speech at the UN and had been staying, under the heaviest security I have ever seen, at the Cuban Mission to the UN, a well-guarded building at 38th and Lex. The security was so tight for Castro that they were having him leave town in the middle of the night.

I realized I might be sitting there for quite some time, so I took evasive action by backing up, making a right on 30th, and cutting across to 1st Avenue, which I used as my route to the bridge. My strategy was successful and I made it over to Queens without further difficulty.

Great! The last thing I needed was to sit in a traffic jam at three in the morning after working an eleven-hour shift. Once over the bridge, I took a couple of side streets to the Long Island Expressway, the quickest route to Forest Hills. I turned on the radio to my favorite station and was on my merry way. I would be home in fifteen minutes. Adios, Manhattan. Adios, Fidel.

But, no.

About a mile after getting on the LIE, there's a merge with the traffic exiting from the Brooklyn–Queens Expressway, the highway I had originally wanted to take. And that is where, once again, the traffic came to a complete stop. In the distance I could see several police cars, lights flashing, blocking the road.

Five minutes went by. Nothing moved. Ten minutes went by. Not an inch. It soon became a surreal kind of scene. Some people were walking around in the middle of the highway, talking to other motorists, others were nodding off in their cars, others tried to keep themselves entertained by listening to their radios. Realizing it had something to do with Castro, I wondered if I would be getting the chance to see him drive by. It might make the ordeal worth it, I thought, if maybe I could make eye contact with Castro and somehow, just by the expression on my face, he'd realize that being a dictator for life was inherently wrong and he'd order free elections as soon as he got back to Cuba. No one would know what had caused him to suddenly embrace democracy, and that would remain a secret just between the two of us.

But, uh, that didn't happen.

What did happen was after nearly an hour, the police cars suddenly turned off their flashing lights and simply drove away. The traffic started moving again. And I got home at around 4.30 a.m.

The next day I read in the paper that Castro had been flown by helicopter from the rooftop of the Cuban Mission to Kennedy Airport. The closing of the BQE and the LIE had been nothing but decoys to confuse a group of Cuban expatriates whom the NYPD apparently had reason to believe would try to assassinate Castro before he left New York.

The 'Get Fidel Out Of New York Alive Traffic Jam' – no, sir, you don't see many of those. Made it into the Hall on the first ballot.

Bad hair day

I found myself driving out to Kew Gardens one evening in 1997 at around seven-thirty with a perfectly nice fellow who didn't want to take the subway home. We were moving along quickly on Queens Boulevard until we were about three-quarters of a mile from his place, and then for reasons unknown the traffic suddenly became completely jammed up and started to crawl at a snail's pace, and a slow snail at that.

After trudging along for ten minutes I could see a multitude of flashing red lights in the distance and I thought it was most likely a serious accident, so after a brief conference with my passenger we decided to take a detour and did some zig-zagging on the back streets to avoid the mess. It was a great move which saved us both some time and probably was the reason for my above-average tip.

After dropping him off I circled around, heading back to Manhattan on the opposite side of Queens Boulevard, and found myself quite near to whatever was going on. Out of natural curiosity I tried to see what was causing the problem, but all I could see were police cars all over the place with their lights flashing. I was ready to forget about it and just get back to Manhattan as quickly as possible when a minor miracle happened – I got a fare back to the city, a middle-aged woman en route to Tribeca.

After the joy of getting this lucky ride subsided, I asked her if she knew what was causing all the excitement on the other side of the boulevard. And, minor miracle number two, she did. I was expecting to hear some story about a gruesome accident or a disturbing crime, but it was neither of those. What she told me was this…

It seems a woman who was an amputee went into a beauty salon to get a new hairdo. She was so displeased with the result that, as a protest against the morons who had done this to her, she decided to take off all her clothes and just sit there. The salon people called the police and when it went out on the radio that a nude female amputee was refusing to put her clothes back on, every patrol car within ten miles responded to the call. So the traffic jam had been caused not by an accident, not by a fire, not by a crime, but by all the cops who, having nowhere else to park their cruisers, just left them on Queens Boulevard and hurried on into the place so they wouldn't miss anything.

Well, of course. *That's* what was causing all the chaos. Why didn't I think of that in the first place? 'The Nude Amputee Traffic Jam' – a connoisseur's delight, and now a proud member of the Traffic Jam Hall of Fame.

So once again we see that making it into the Hall is not just a matter of size nor of the amount of time it consumes. It must be unique, caused by something we've never seen before, something we never would have suspected.

Something like *this*…

After a good meal

At around 9.30 p.m. on December 16, 1985, I stopped for a woman with two large boxes at Bond Street and the Bowery in the East Village. I got out of the cab to deposit the boxes in the trunk and we were soon on our way to her destination, 54th Street between 2nd and 3rd Avenues. The Bowery changes its name to 3rd Avenue just a few blocks up the road, so this was going to be a straight run uptown to 54th with only one turn at the end. It was navigation in its most basic form.

By 9.30 the evening rush hour has been over for more than an hour and if you're going to hit any traffic at all on 3rd Avenue, it will be up in the fifties as you approach the 59th Street Bridge. So we were both quite surprised when the traffic slowed to a crawl at 32nd Street. Immediately the conjecture began.

What could it be?

A problem on the FDR Drive, causing an overflow of cars to exit at 34th Street? Possibly, but unlikely because if that were the case most of the traffic would be on 1st Avenue, not as far away from the FDR as 3rd.

Roadwork? Always a possibility, but we could see the traffic was backed up on 3rd as far as the eye could see, and roadwork didn't usually back things up that much, at least not at that time of the evening.

Christmas traffic? No way, we were much too far away from Rockefeller Center, the source of all Christmas woes.

So what *could* it be? We didn't know, but after seven or eight minutes of progressing only a couple of blocks, our thoughts turned to taking a detour. We could make a left on 35th and take Park Avenue up to 54th, or we could turn right on 36th and take 1st. I was about to suggest that we should take Park when the traffic suddenly started moving a bit. We trudged along at five miles per hour for a few blocks, giving us hope that the jam was ending, but our hopes were dashed when we got to 38th Street and it froze up again. And to add to our misery, we could see way up the avenue that there was police activity in progress. An experienced eye can tell the magnitude of the event by the brightness of the flashing lights, which gives you an idea of how many emergency vehicles are on the scene. And I judged that this one was major.

It looked like the lights were about six or seven blocks away, and the question again was do we or do we not turn off 3rd and take an alternate route. Considering that the cause of the problem was in sight, we agreed that the right thing to do was just to stay the course. Unfortunately for both of us, the option of my passenger getting out and walking the rest of the way was not to be considered, since she had the two large boxes in the trunk. So on we went. Or maybe I should say, on we crawled, because it took another ten or twelve minutes to finally reach the exact spot that was causing the whole mess.

And that spot was on 46th Street, where the entire avenue, except for one lane on the left, was filled with police cars, ambulances, and about a dozen media trucks with their satellite antennas sticking into the air like high-tech mechanical swords. At the one open lane, with all the traffic filtering into it, stood a solitary cop trying to keep things moving with a waving arm. And as we finally merged into the lane, we heard him saying these immortal words:

'Mafia hit, keep it moving. Mafia hit, keep it moving.'

Paul Castellano, a Mafia boss, had been gunned down as he exited Sparks Steak House on 46th between 2nd and 3rd. *That* was the cause of the traffic jam. (It's the luckiest thing that can happen to a restaurant in New York, by the way, as it guarantees business for years to come. The owner of a bistro down the block was quoted in the papers the next day moaning, 'If I'd only had time, I would have dragged the body in front of my *own* place!')

Yes, 'The Mafia Hit Traffic Jam', an exotic item indeed and a unanimous choice for membership in the Hall.

Benvenuto!

15

Solids, Liquids and Gases

I had just started driving a night shift on a Sunday in March, 1994, and soon found myself sitting in the taxi line in front of Macy's awaiting the arrival of my first customer of the evening. After a couple of minutes a woman came out of the 'World's Largest Store', as the gigantic sign at the corner of 34th Street and Broadway proclaims, and sat herself down in the back seat. She told me her destination, I pulled out from the taxi stand, drove half a block, and stopped at a red light at 34th. Suddenly she opened her door, stepped out onto the pavement, and slammed the door shut.

'Someone has *urinated* in this taxi!' she screamed in complete disgust and then stomped off in search of another, less offensive cab.

I had detected an errant odor when I'd left the garage, but hadn't been able to put my finger on exactly what it was and then started the shift kind of hoping no one would notice. So much for that idea.

Matter comes to us in three forms: solids, liquids and gases. The taxicab is not immune to the trouble these forms may create and any cabbie has a particular dread of their tendency to go astray. So serious is this dread that I have surmised that the four worst things that can happen to a cab driver are:

1. Death

2. Paralysis

3. Armed robbery

4. Some subhuman pukes in your cab.

Puke, that most vile of all human liquids, belongs in the digestive tract well concealed and well contained, a law that is fundamental to all civilizations since the beginning of time. Consider the horror of discovering that your passenger does not feel a need to abide by this basic tenet. First, you must somehow force yourself not to kill him. Second, you must scream at him. Third, you've got to demand that he pay you for the misery he has caused (London cabs, the world's elite, have a 'soiling charge' which requires offenders to pay for their crime. There's no such thing in New York City). Fourth, when you see he's not going to pay, you've got to demand that he clean it up himself. Fifth, when you finally realize he's a semi-coherent slab of meat that is not capable of cleaning it up himself, you've got to curse him out as you begin to drive back to your garage to get Antonio to clean it up for you. Sixth, you've got to pay Antonio ten bucks to do the job.

Dealing with this runaway liquid is as bad as it gets. All right, death, paralysis and a gun pointed at the back of your head – as listed above – would be worse, but that's it! Aside from the time and money lost, there is the sheer insult of it. It's as if the passenger is saying to you, 'I'm going to throw up now, but I'm not going to bother telling you that I'm about to do it so you can pull over and let me barf out there on the street. I'm not even going to stick my head out the window. No, what I'm going to do is just puke right here in your cab. That way, when I'm done, you can clean it up yourself and then work with the smell for the rest of your shift. Oh, and by the way, have a nice night.'

Really, what could be more insulting than that?

So any cab driver develops a built-in alarm system for the danger of the potential puker. It turns out there are two basic types: a) the sick, and b) the drunk. Oddly enough, the sick are the ones who provoke the most anger in the driver. That's because although they may be ill, they are sober. Which means they're aware of what they're doing.

I once had a twenty-something guy as my first passenger on a Wednesday evening in September, 1997, who was en route to Queens from Times Square – just a normal-looking fellow apparently going home from work. As we were approaching the 59th Street Bridge I became aware of an odd, apple-like odor in the taxi. My antennas went up.

'There's a weird smell in here. Did you just *throw up*?' I asked with considerable anxiety.

'No,' he replied innocently.

We drove another block and stopped for a red light. The smell had gotten stronger, so I turned around and took a look in the back. He was just sitting there with puke all over himself and the seat.

'Jesus Christ!' I screamed.

'I'm sick,' he moaned.

I wasn't moved to pity. Too sick to let me know what was going on so I could let him out and let him do it in the street? No. I flew into a rage and then, barely able to contain myself from adding 'broken nose' to his health problems, I deposited him right there on 59th Street and headed back to the garage.

To Antonio.

The drunks, however, far outnumber the sick and are therefore the greatest risk, especially on a Friday night and especially, *especially* on a Saturday night, which might as well just be called 'drunk night' in New York City. A veteran cabbie driving on those nights is constantly on the alert for the vomit candidate, always looking for the signs.

Signs like difficulty opening the door, too much time trying to tell you where in the hell he's going, muttering noises which turn out to be the guy talking to himself when you were hoping he was on his cell phone, odd laughter for no reason whatsoever, opening his window, and, most ominous of all, his head disappears from the rearview mirror and you find he has slumped over on his side in a semi-conscious stupor.

You've got to keep your eye on the passenger who has any of these signs in order to figure out just how likely it is that he may indeed soon be emptying the contents of his stomach all over the back seat. It's as if there's a 'vomit warning' light flashing on the dashboard – now *there's* something that should be standard equipment in any taxi!

Handling this person is as delicate an operation as walking on a tightrope with a clown – one false move and you've had it. The first thing you need to do is to decide if you should even ask them if they're feeling sick. With some of them, you have a sense that doing so will by itself *cause* them to puke, like a hypnotic suggestion. If it seems safe to proceed, you've got to try to minimize the risk by giving them a little speech that goes something like this:

Driver: 'How are you feeling?'

Passenger: 'Okay.'

Driver: 'Tell me the truth, now – are you feeling like you might be sick?'

Passenger: 'I don't know… a little, maybe… I'll be okay.'

Driver: (Looking him right in the eye) 'Okay, here's the deal. It's *very important* that you don't puke in my cab. You understand that? If you feel like you're going to be sick, *tell me*, and I'll pull over to the side of the road. Are we cool on this?'

It doesn't really matter what he says. You just feel that laying down the law is the least you can do to try to ward off disaster. Then the ride begins. And the tension mounts.

What you resist

She came out of a club in Times Square on a Saturday night at 4 a.m. and wanted to go way out to Bay Ridge, Brooklyn, a thirty-minute ride. She was a club-age girl (in her early twenties) and I could tell merely from the way she said hello that she was a nice kid without an attitude who just needed to get home after a long night of partying. The timing of the ride was tight but doable for me. My shift ends at 5 a.m. and I would have just about enough time to get her to Bay Ridge, gas up the cab, and get back to my garage on the west side of Manhattan.

So we were on our way.

Within two blocks she showed the first sign of trouble by rolling down her window on what was a cold, November night.

Uh-oh. An inexperienced driver might ignore this, but, as you know, I don't. I didn't think bringing up the subject would do any damage, so I gave her the you-mustn't-puke-in-my-cab speech, nicely, and discovered that she was, indeed, feeling 'a bit' nauseous. Although I didn't show it, I immediately felt the same kind of panic you get when you find yourself suddenly losing control of your car on an icy road. Plus, I had a problem.

The problem was that I wanted the cash for the ride, but at the same time I wanted to get rid of her. However, I had no viable justification for doing so. She was alert and coherent. She knew where she wanted to go and could even help me with directions if I needed them. Plus she was a nice person. So I was stuck with her and decided to plow on through.

We headed down Broadway toward the Brooklyn Bridge.

After establishing the extreme importance of not vomiting in the cab, the next thing to do is to keep your eye continually on the passenger. Just because they say they're going to tell you to pull over doesn't mean they will. And finally, you must keep them talking. All the way. Create a world between just the two of you where vomit doesn't exist and don't let them slip away to a place where the demons of regurgitation can whisper in their ear.

So chit-chat we did.

We talked about the club she'd been in, we talked about the rain; we talked about the price of tea in Chinatown, we talked about Spain. We talked about the things she used to do when she was a child; we talked about Oscar de la Renta and Oscar de la Wilde. In short, we talked about anything I could think of to keep her attention away from puking.

And it seemed to be working just fine until I turned onto Duane Street, just a couple of blocks from the bridge. Suddenly she stopped talking. Looking at her in the mirror, she appeared to be trying to hold it in.

Oh, shit.

'How are you doing, there?' asked I.

There was a pause. And then, finally…

'Uhh… I'm feelin' kinda sick.'

Have you ever heard that expression about the driver who 'stopped on a dime'? Well, I don't know if there was a dime out there on Duane Street, but if there was, I certainly stopped on it, bringing the taxi to an abrupt and definitive halt.

'Please, miss, step outside the cab!'

Fortunately she was the compliant type. Some people are too embarrassed to stand out in the street and throw up in full view of the world (but not too embarrassed to do it in a taxicab). Like a good soldier, she opened the door, stumbled out onto the street, and positioned herself between two parked cars for 'privacy', and let it fly. I gave her some paper towels as she returned to the cab.

'Feeling better?'

'Yes, thank you, a lot better.'

I breathed the proverbial sigh of relief. A crisis that had been feared had come to pass, but we had made it through without catastrophe. If this had been a movie, it would have been the part where the hero (me) was about to live happily ever after. All was right with the world again.

Our chit-chat returned.

I made a right on Broadway, a left on Chambers, and we were soon on the stately and perhaps it would not be an exaggeration to say *magnificent* Brooklyn Bridge, the prototype for the steel-wire suspension bridge and one of New York's great sights. And it was immediately after I asked her if she knew that the construction of the bridge had been completed before the invention of the automobile that I became alarmed by a new pause in our conversation. She was staring blankly at the space just in front of her and not commenting on my question. This was *not good*!

'Are you all right?' I inquired, already knowing she wasn't.

'I, uh, I don't know… I think I might be feeling sick again…'

A wave of desperation gripped me, worse than before – because *you can't stop on the bridge!* I felt like I was dangling from a rope and was about to fall into an East River of puke.

'I can't stop on the bridge!' I called out to her.

Looking in the mirror, I could see that she was in a mighty struggle to keep it inside her body and I remembered reading somewhere that you can get rid of hiccups by extroverting the attention of the afflicted, so the thought occurred to me that maybe I ought to try to get her to sing. Nobody pukes while they're singing, right? So I did an instant mental scan for the right song and came up with 'A Hundred Bottles of Beer on the Wall', something we could sing together and would keep her counting. Then I looked at her again in the mirror and saw that she was sitting with her head quite close to the opened window – the prepared-to-puke position – and realized that the idea of a sing-along, particularly to a song with bottles of beer in the lyrics, was perhaps the stupidest idea I'd had since I decided to purchase a beat-up cab from the owner of a taxi garage for use as my own car.

There seemed to be only one thing to do, and that was to step on the gas and get off the bridge as fast as I possibly could. I called into the back to offer encouragement.

'Listen,' I shouted, 'try to hold it in, but if you can't, do it out the window! I'll pull over as soon as we're off the bridge! Okay?'

She nodded agreement and I went into NASCAR mode, deftly bolting around the cars around me like the chase scene in a movie. It was the kind of driving that requires you to keep your eyes completely focused on the road ahead, so I couldn't even glance in the mirror to see how she was doing. Instead, I resigned myself to the probability that the rear door, inside and out, and the rear fender were about to get a vomit bath. These out-the-window pukers never get it all out onto the street, especially at high speeds. Still, it was better than coming down on the seat or the floorboard, so I could count that as a blessing of sorts.

I roared out of there, nearly clipping a Volkswagen Beetle as I executed a double-lane turn at the first exit off the bridge, and brought the cab to a stop as soon as I was away from the flow of traffic. With great anticipation, I turned and looked to see what damage had been done. And to my great surprise, there was nothing!

She was just sitting there, composed and almost serene, it seemed, as if she'd been enjoying the ride and the snap of the cool night air.

'How are you?' I asked.

'I'm okay,' she replied.

'Oh… *good*!' I said, somewhat amazed. 'Well, let's go to Bay Ridge. Let me know, you know, if you start feeling sick again.'

'I will, don't worry.'

I pulled out into the traffic and realized immediately that I had a new, tough decision to make. The entrance to the Brooklyn–Queens Expressway, the highway that would take us to Bay Ridge, was only a few blocks away. The travel time would be about eight minutes, assuming there were no traffic problems, something that can always happen on that road, even at four in the morning. The problem was that the BQE is an expressway with very few shoulder areas, thus there would be *no place to pull over* should she get sick again. However, we could take the side streets, although it would add precious minutes to the ride.

I had to make up my mind immediately. I looked in the mirror at the human time bomb sitting in the back seat. Then I looked at my own mental image of a scowling Steve, the night dispatcher at my garage, as I brought the cab in late.

I opted for the side streets. To hell with Steve.

I told her my plan. She was fine with it and told me again that she was feeling okay now. Still, to be on the safe side, I wanted the side streets. She said okay. I bypassed the entrance to the BQE, made a left on Furman Street, and we were on our way once again.

After driving for about a minute I felt I should keep the conversation going, so I asked her how she liked living in Bay Ridge. She replied that she liked it fine. I mentioned that the iconic film character 'Tony Manero', played by John Travolta in *Saturday Night Fever*, was supposed to have lived in Bay Ridge and, amazingly, I once had a woman in my cab who lived in Bay Ridge in real life who said during the ride that her own last name was 'Manero'!

'Was that incredible, or what?' I called into the back. 'I mean, it was almost enough to make you start thinking *everyone* in Bay Ridge must be named "Manero"! Right? Hey, *your* last name isn't "Manero", is it?'

I looked at her in the mirror hoping to see an amused expression on her face, but instead what I saw was that same look of anxiety, her head once again tilting close to the opened window. There was no killing this thing.

'You're feeling sick again?'

'Yeah...'

I hit the brakes and stopped. Knowing the drill by now, she promptly stepped out of the cab, hunched herself over, and after a few tentative spasms, added a bit more puke to the city streets. I handed her another paper towel as she got back in the cab and she accepted it with a barely audible 'thanks', as if this whole thing was becoming an expected and acceptable routine.

I congratulated myself in my own thoughts for being so perceptive and downright brilliant about choosing the side streets over the highway. Had we been on the BQE, that puke would have been all over my door and things would have been so much worse not only due to the indignity of having to clean up another person's vomit, but also because that clean-up would have put an additional delay on bringing the cab back to the garage. If you come in too far beyond the 5 a.m. shift end-time and the day driver has been caused to wait for the cab, thus losing time he has paid for, he would be within his rights to demand compensation. And how miserable would that be? You drive for twelve hours non-stop on a Saturday night, putting up with all kinds of drunks, you wind up cleaning up some moron's vomit *and then you have to pay another driver for the time it took to clean that vomit up.*

No, no, *noooooo*!

We drove on. With the delays we'd already had, the time factor was becoming more important in my mind. Then, as we approached the next entrance to the BQE at Atlantic Avenue, Navigation Dilemma Number Two begged for my attention. Should I now get off the side streets and get on the highway? Was she all puked out? I looked at her again in the mirror. She seemed fine, but what did that prove? This girl was a puke machine. Still, I thought that after three heaves she couldn't really have any more left in the tank. Then I thought again of Steve. Then I thought of the angry day driver demanding twenty bucks for his lost time.

I got on the ramp leading to the highway.

'Listen, I'm gettin' on the BQE,' I said. 'You're okay, now, right?'

'Yeah, I'm okay.'

'Okay, so listen, if you feel sick again, you'll have to put it out the window. Okay?'

'Don't worry. I'm fine now.'

'Okay.'

I got on the BQE and stepped on the gas. Although I was flying, there was much more wiggle room on the BQE than there had been on the Brooklyn Bridge, so I could glance at her in the mirror occasionally. And she seemed fine. We chatted a bit about Bay Ridge and other places she had lived, but for the most part I just kept my attention on the road and drove as quickly as safety would allow. In five minutes we were exiting the expressway, and in two more minutes we were sitting in front of her apartment building.

She apologized for the condition she was in and the trouble it had caused me. I said not to be concerned, I had enjoyed chatting with her. She paid me the fare and tipped well above average. We exchanged goodbyes and she disappeared into her building. I drove down to the end of the block and stopped at a red light. And then it hit me.

This thing had ended too well. Maybe she had puked when I wasn't looking. Maybe her generous tip had been given to ease her conscience because she knew she was leaving me a 'souvenir'. I decided to take a good look in the back. Fearing the worst, I:

- put the cab in 'park',
- stepped out onto the street,
- opened the rear door,
- confronted Fate,
- and looked.

And what do you know, there was nothing! My outlook on life, taxi driving and Steve immediately changed for the better. Happiness, it turns out, is a clean seat.

And so, with this new, optimistic point of view, I headed back to Manhattan and the taxi garage. The clock on my dashboard was now at 4.35 a.m., so returning on time, or at least close to on time, did not appear to be a problem. I got back on the BQE and by 4.50 a.m. I was cruising up Hudson Street in lower Manhattan, heading toward the Hess gas station at 45th and 10th.

Now, if you drive the night shift on Saturday, there's a lovely phenomenon that occurs between 4.30 and 5.30 a.m.. At the same time that the taxi shift is ending, thus creating a shortage of available cabs, all the clubs are letting out, thus creating a surplus of customers. So a driver, trying to make a few extra dollars, can take his pick from dozens of stranded club people who are milling around on the streets. The way to do it correctly is to a) put on your 'off-duty' light, b) lock the doors, and c) approach a person on the street slowly and call out to him that you can only do a short ride. That way you avoid a trip that would cause you to be late getting back to the garage, plus you make extra cash.

Using this time-tested technique, I spotted a twenty-something fellow with his hand in the air at Leroy and Hudson. He told me he wanted to go to 54th between 9th and 10th in Hell's Kitchen. It was a perfect, going-my-way ride, free money and a cherry on the top of the cake that had been my shift. He got in and we headed uptown.

I didn't try to make any conversation with this guy. He'd be in and out in five minutes and, truth be told, I viewed him as just a bit of cargo I was transporting on a route I would have taken anyway. He was literally just along for the ride and he didn't appear to be the chatty type, anyway. So, other than the sound of the music on my radio, it was a silent ride, but what mattered most was that it was a fast ride. By 4.58 he'd been dropped off at his place on 54th Street and I was $10 richer. And heading for the Hess station.

Taxi drivers who lease cabs from taxi garages are responsible for filling the cab with gasoline before returning it to the garage. That way the next driver starts his shift with a full tank. So when I arrived at the Hess station, which is very busy at that time of the night, I went into my end-of-shift routine. Aside from filling the cab with gas, that routine includes cleaning out any garbage that had accumulated during the shift from both myself in the front and the passengers in the rear. My own stuff in the front tends to be the same every night: about twenty receipt papers that had not been taken by passengers (they come out of the meter automatically at the end of every ride) and remnants of the food I'd eaten during the course of the shift. The stuff in the rear, however, tends to be much more interesting. You never know what you may find back there – aside from discarded papers and cigarette butts, there's always the chance you may discover something of value, like money.

Knowing this, there's just a touch of anticipation when opening that rear door. *Will I find a wallet? A cell phone? Some cash? How about a hundred dollar bill?* (It happened once.) It's kind of like a quiz show – '*and now... behind Door Number Three...* (drum roll)...'

How about a seat covered with puke?

Yes, that is what I found when I opened that door – *a seat covered with puke!* What I had made such great efforts to avoid during the trip to Bay Ridge had come to pass during the silent ride with that last passenger, to whom I had paid no attention whatsoever.

Several minutes of cursing, wailing and cursing again at whatever Force was following me around and toying with me eventually subsided and gave way to a contemplation of this interesting philosophical truism: *that what you resist, you become.*

Isn't that the truth? Try just a little too hard to avoid falling on your butt and there he is, Fate's little messenger boy, going unnoticed in the crowd, dropping banana peels in front of you on the sidewalk.

Well, I'm sure you can now appreciate the stress, if not outright horror, that a taxi driver endures when liquids go astray. Aside from puke and urine, as we've touched on, let's not forget spit, snot, a whitish substance you hope is not sperm, soft drinks, beer, milk and paint. Yes, *paint* – it happened to me once. The passenger was a professional sign painter and knocked over a can of paint with his knee. Now you know why the interiors of New York City taxicabs are always made of vinyl (waterproof).

Let's move on to a form of matter that, although less insidious, is nevertheless a cause for great concern – *gases.* No, not the kind they sell at the Hess station. If I may be candid for a moment, ladies and gentlemen, we're about to delve into the unspeakable subjects of flatulence and body odor. In my capacity as the Complaint Department for the entire taxi industry in New York City, second only to the rants I have to listen to about drivers who can't speak English are the rants I have to listen to about drivers who stink.

'Don't these guys know what deodorant is?' a passenger wails.

'I guess it's a cultural thing,' I reply.

The problem originates from the grim reality that a driver must sit in an enclosed space for as long as twelve hours and his body, like the car he drives, has its own exhaust system. Aside from Speed Stick by Mennen, Old Spice, and those air fresheners that look like pine trees, I have discovered that the best handling of this problem can be described in one word – 'ventilation'. Advice to drivers: those buttons on the armrest are there for a reason. Open the windows!

One of the cruelest jokes ever perpetuated on the human race by the industrial age, by the way, is the catalytic converter that is going bad. The catalytic converter is a device in the exhaust system of modern cars that prevents environmentally harmful gases from entering the atmosphere. When they start to go bad they may emit a rotten egg odor which can travel into the interior of the cab. So a comical situation can occur in which both the passenger and the driver think that the other is a social Neanderthal, having passed gas in a shared space. Who would believe that the actual culprit was the car?

Now, it should be noted that not *all* smells in taxicabs are repugnant. For one thing, if you should be lucky enough to be a passenger in a new cab, there is that 'new car' smell. Everybody loves that. Then there's the 'perfume hour', from 7 to 8 p.m. It's the time of the evening when the majority of people who are going out for the night are on their way to wherever they're going and the scents they may have added to their bodies are at top strength. That's usually a pleasant experience. Add to these the various aromas of hot foods that people carry into cabs, such as pizza, coffee and bagfuls of burgers and fries, and you can find yourself in an olfactory wonderland, a place inhabited by a remarkable passenger I had in my cab one night.

Bloodhound

He was a normal-looking thirty-something who jumped in at around 2 a.m. in Midtown, heading up to 85th and Columbus on the Upper West Side. As we crossed from 6th Avenue to 8th on 43rd Street, it was becoming what I would call a 'comfortable' ride. He was a pleasant person, easy to talk to, and we became engaged in a lively conversation, moving effortlessly from sports to local politics. Then, about ten minutes into it, without the slightest provocation, he uttered this total non sequitur:

'Sesame bagel.'

'Sesame bagel?' I repeated back to him. 'What do you mean, "sesame bagel"?'

'Someone ate a sesame bagel in here.' It wasn't a question. It was a statement.

'Why? Are there remnants of a bagel on the floor back there?'

'No, I can smell it.'

I could smell nothing of the sort and didn't know what he was talking about. Then it hit me – *I* had eaten a sesame bagel in the cab at nine o'clock that evening, *five hours earlier!* My nightly routine included taking a break at a place called 'Hot Bagels' on 2nd Avenue and 35th Street and grabbing a bagel and a cup of coffee, which I consumed when I continued driving. All that was left of it were a few crumbs and sesame seeds that were wrapped up in a squashed paper bag located in the sleeve of my door, where I store my trash until the end of the shift.

It turned out the guy had a superhuman sense of smell, like a dog. It was a rare condition, he said, the medical name for which was 'hyperosmia'. He said he'd only ever heard of one other person who was known to have it, as well.

You may hear or read about people from time to time who are said to have superhuman abilities, but it is next to never that you actually get to witness one in action with your own eyes (or nose). To this day I count this little incident as one of the most remarkable things I have ever observed first hand.

It makes you wonder, though, what the guy's life must be like. Yikes! If I had my choice of superhuman abilities, I think I'd choose gargantuan strength. The kind of strength that would enable me to lift a car into the air with one hand. Or to easily extricate an unconscious, two hundred and fifty pound man from the back seat of my cab.

Which brings us to *solids.*

There are certain rides that start out with a mobile human being lumbering into the back seat and end with an unconscious meaty hulk that cannot be communicated with nor moved – a solid. Assuming the body is still breathing, what has happened here is that the driver has made the mistake of letting someone get into his cab who was *too* drunk in the first place. Once the ride begins, the alcohol further kicks in and the passenger slumps over in a boozy coma. The important thing to do, if you suspect this may happen, is to get paid and get an exact address of his destination before the ride begins. Otherwise you may find yourself with a body and a problem.

I once made the mistake of accepting a ride with the vague address of 'Bayside', a far-off section of Queens, from a young man who'd just emerged from a private party at Ferrier, a chic East Side restaurant which, he mentioned, had accommodated him with an open bar. By the time we were over the Queensborough Bridge the guy had disappeared from my rearview mirror and was unresponsive to questions about where, exactly, he lived. I just drove on, figuring he'd awaken from his dreams by the time we arrived in Bayside. Instead, all my shouting, clapping, banging against the partition, and shaking of his arms could not produce the slightest response. Finally I tracked down a squad car and, miraculously, the guy awakened by some magical ability cops must have to arouse the dead. I eventually did get him to his home, but found when we got there that in his stupor he no longer knew who I was nor why he was in my car. Several theater-of-the-absurd minutes later I was able to convince him that I was his taxi driver, but he was only able to come up with half of what was on the meter – which I gladly accepted just to get rid of him.

So you see what a problem these solids can be.

But, you know, there is one way of handling a problem that has been part of the human race's bag of tricks since the wheel was invented – and then broke. And that is to give the problem to someone else.

The drunk drop

In all team sports there are certain set plays that are used as part of a strategy in trying to win the game. In baseball, for example, there's a play called the 'suicide squeeze'. In American football there's the 'down and out'. In basketball they have one called the 'pick and roll'.

In taxi driving, there's the 'drunk drop'.

The drunk drop is when a patron of a bar or restaurant has become so drunk that he or she is semi-coherent and is bordering on becoming incoherent or even passing out completely (a solid). The patron is then escorted, hustled or just carried from the establishment by bartenders or waiters and is deposited into a taxicab. If the taxi drives away, the strategy has been successful. The drunk has been 'dropped' and is now somebody else's problem.

One evening in May, 2008, I was cruising down 2nd Avenue on the Upper East Side at around 9 p.m., looking for my next fare. As I passed 89th Street someone with his hand in the air appeared from the left side of the avenue, so I deftly cut over and pulled to a stop. There's great craft in being able to cut through traffic safely and swiftly, but there's also great craft in being able to instantly size a person up before you allow them access into your vehicle. And in this I was lacking.

As I stopped my cab what I saw approaching from the curb were three people – two men in waiter's attire flanking a middle-aged woman, a blonde, and kind of half-carrying her. In other words she was walking on her own volition, but just barely, and the men had their arms under her arms to catch her should she stumble or fall.

It was a drunk drop in progress.

Normally if I see it coming I either keep on driving or, if I'm already at a stop, I lock the doors. But perhaps due to my reflexes slowing down with age, or for whatever reason, I just froze there for a moment. And that moment was all that was needed for one of the waiters to get his hand on the door and open it.

And in came the drunk.

The waiters then turned around and walked back into their restaurant, a chic little Mediterranean joint. One of them said something to the other that made him laugh.

For just a second I let myself think that maybe she'd just turned her ankle or something and wasn't actually drunk at all. Maybe she just needed some help walking and I'd probably be driving her to the emergency room of a hospital. But one look at her as she plopped down on the seat with her head tilted to the side told me that was just wishful thinking.

I asked her where she wanted to go. There was a long pause. I repeated the question. Finally she said, rather conclusively…

'I don't know.'

Yes, not only did she not know where she wanted to go, she was *sure* she didn't know where she wanted to go. But at least she could respond to a question, even if it took half a minute to do so. That was a plus. After another futile attempt to get a destination out of her, I realized I had to pull a play of my own…

The Reverse Drunk Drop

It's a wise cabbie who realizes that he mustn't step on the gas pedal in a situation like this. There is potential trouble in all directions here, especially if the semi-coherent inebriate is a female. So the play is to reverse the drop that has given you the drunk. Or, to put it in postal terms, 'Return To Sender'.

I got out of my cab, leaving the woman in the back, and walked into the restaurant. The two waiters were nowhere in sight, but a fellow who looked like he was some kind of a maitre d' was standing there. I told him in a voice that was calm yet had an element of restrained anger in it that two waiters from his restaurant had just put a woman in my cab who was so drunk that she couldn't so much as tell me where she wanted to go. And that they'd better come back and get her out of my cab.

Or I would call the police.

And with that I turned around and walked out of the place.

I returned to my cab, opened the rear door, and confronted the unwanted cargo that was sitting there. She had opened her bag and was looking through the objects in it, apparently hoping to find a clue as to what her destination might be. I was searching for a way to tell her that she was too wasted to meet the minimum requirements for membership in my club when I was confronted myself by one of the waiters who had dumped her there, and he wasn't too happy with the situation.

I was perfectly willing to handle the matter in a civil tone, but the guy, a slightly built man in his forties who was a bit shorter than I, was in a non-negotiating, attack mode. Immediately he was yelling at me, demanding to know who the hell I thought I was, walking into his restaurant like I was some kind of authority, the implication being that taxi drivers should be seen and not heard.

Well, I don't want to use profane language to describe this guy, so instead of saying what kind of hole he appeared to be, I'll just say that he closely resembled an orifice that is found at the very end of the alimentary canal. What followed was one of those scenes that seem comical in retrospect, but in the moment are red-hot episodes of human idiocy.

The waiter got right in my face, allowing for only about an inch of space between us and also providing me with an opportunity to learn that he'd been sampling the garlic bread in the kitchen. With a 'how dare you?' this and a 'the nerve of you' that, he flew into a self-righteous rage which would have given the passerby on the street the impression that *I* was the offending party.

Of course, it was all pretense. This phony was trying to deflect attention away from his own misdeeds. When people have secrets you're a bit too close to discovering, they have a definite tendency to become quite upset with you, and the neon sign that announces this is their self-righteous indignation.

One secret he had, no doubt, was that he'd served the woman far too many drinks. This could be a big problem to the owner of the restaurant, and thus to the waiter, as it could lead to the revocation of their liquor license if harm should come to her as a result. And there may have been other things he didn't want revealed, as well. Perhaps he'd lifted money from her purse after she'd been reduced to a semi-conscious blob. Perhaps he'd overcharged her. Perhaps he'd decided to give himself a $50 tip when he ran her credit card through the system.

Of course, I didn't know what it was, but I did know it was something. And what I also knew was that this guy's aggression toward me was about to become a shoving match. And that could lead to a punching match. And that could lead to – well, it could lead to a very bad night, indeed.

But then, as often happens in life – at least in my life, it seems – a sort of divine intervention occurred.

In a scene that was reminiscent of something you might see in a silent movie, the woman suddenly emerged from the back seat of the cab, took a couple of wobbly steps forward, and then fell straight down like a sack of blonde potatoes onto the pavement.

There was a sudden break in the action.

The waiter looked at the woman.

The waiter looked at me.

The waiter looked back at the woman.

What to do???

Fortunately, the waiter went with the woman. He dropped his 'you wanna fight, taxi-schmuck?' demeanor and with a new demeanor of frustrated desperation began attending to his fallen customer, first lifting her up and then guiding her into one of the seats on the sidewalk in front of his restaurant.

Thus the Reverse Drunk Drop was ruled by the imaginary referee I carry around with me to be an official success. I got back in my cab and called 911 on my cell phone, telling them there was a semi-coherent woman who needed assistance in front of this particular establishment.

They said they'd send an ambulance.

And that was good enough for me.

I took off down 2nd Avenue in search of my next fare with thoughts of drunk drops past and present dancing through my mind. And wondering what in the hell my next out-of-nowhere adventure might be. Which, to tell you the truth, is the best part of being a taxi driver.

[illegible]

[illegible]

[illegible]

There was a [illegible]

The [illegible]

The [illegible]

[illegible]

[illegible]

[illegible]

[illegible]

[illegible]

Then [illegible]

And [illegible]

And the [illegible]

16

'Taxi!'

How do you get a cab in New York City? You *hail* it.

> Hail (verb) - to attract the attention of through motions or calls: Let's hail a taxi.
> (*Macmillan Dictionary for Students*)

It may not have occurred to many that the hail is a form of human communication that is unique to only a few cities in the world. In Manhattan, due to the density of the population, it's a workable system by which to obtain the service of a taxicab. In one of the other boroughs, like Staten Island, however, it wouldn't work so well because people are too spread out to make cruising the streets practical – a cabbie would be spinning his wheels on relatively empty streets. So in most areas of the world, taxis depend on a two-way radio system to get their business.

In New York, however, the 13,237 yellow cabs don't use radios to find passengers. In fact, since the mid-'80s they have been forbidden. There are many thousands of community car service vehicles in the boroughs and corporate 'black cars' in Manhattan that do have radios, but the yellow cabs get all their business from street hails and airport rides.

So a cabbie becomes quite expert at recognizing when someone on the street is not just someone raising his hand to scratch his head, but is actually trying to obtain his services. It's as if he has a radar that is perpetually scanning the streets in search of that next customer. And one thing he discovers before too long is that there are varying degrees of proficiency in the way people execute 'the hail'. Some are amazingly good at it, while others need to practice, practice, *practice*! It's a skill.

Tourists are usually from places where there is no such thing as a street hail, so, like any novice, they haven't yet learned the right way to go about it. Whenever you see someone standing on the sidewalk and waving his hand at a taxi, for example, you know it's a tourist. New Yorkers are *always* a few steps out onto the street, knowing instinctively that they need to make themselves visible to approaching cabs.

A few years after becoming a cab driver and witnessing many thousands of hails, I began to feel a need to start judging them. 'Wow, that was a good one!' I would think after seeing a woman march out of Bloomingdale's and get my attention with merely the flick of her hand. Or, 'Ouch!' I would moan as I realized, looking through the rearview mirror, that the person I had just driven by had actually been trying to hail me and had *not* been rubbing his nose. As more years went by I became dissatisfied with merely rating hails as 'good' or 'bad' and sought to improve upon my method of judgment. And thus *The International Taxi-Hailing Point System* was born, a system by which we can acknowledge those who do it well and castigate those who do it poorly.

How do you judge a hail? Well, there are two general areas to be considered: *technique* and *style.* Both are equally important in awarding a fair score to the would-be passenger. Let's take a look at these.

Technique is simply the ability to communicate to the cab driver that his service is desired. It's just a basic thing – was the prospective passenger effective in getting across this message from Point A (himself) to Point B (the cabbie)?

Style is the flair with which that communication is accomplished. It's an aesthetic thing.

In awarding a score, both technique and style are considered separately and equally. The scale used is from 1.0 (abysmally bad) to 6.0 (perfect), as in ice skating.

Example: a middle-aged female Workerbee, dressed for business, is standing near the intersection of 39th and 5th, looking for a cab. She positions herself on the street, only a foot away from the curb. As an available cab is approaching, she looks at the cab, does *not* make eye contact with the driver, and initiates her hail only when the cab is just a quarter of a block in front of her. She then raises her arm only halfway up, leaving her elbow bent, and continues to hold her arm that way for a full second after the taxi has come to a halt. Finally she examines the driver for a moment before opening the door and getting in.

How do we rate this hail? First, let's look at her technique.

She *did* attract the attention of the cab driver and get the cab to stop for her. This is important, and she has so far received no deductions. However, she was too close to the curb, making it difficult for the driver to notice her. For this blunder a full point is deducted, as visibility is the most basic element of the hail. Furthermore, she waited too long before raising her hand, not giving the driver enough time to make a smooth approach and thus causing him to brake hard as he pulled over to her. Another point is deducted for this error, giving her a score of 4.0 for technique.

Now let's look at her style.

The scoring for style takes into consideration the character of the person who is hailing. It should fit the persona of that individual and the situation that individual is in. In this case we see a middle-aged woman in business attire and expect her hail to reflect a person who has had some experience in life and is relatively efficient in the way she goes about things. She should have known better than to be too close to the curb, so she loses a style point there. Her failure to make eye contact with the driver shows a thoughtlessness out of character. Deduct half a point. Her keeping her hand in the air after the cab had stopped demonstrates a failure to observe what is happening. Very bad form, indeed, deduct a full point. And her examining the cabbie before getting in the cab indicates a distrust inappropriate for a seasoned business person, thus causing the loss of another half-point and giving her a final score of 3.5 for style.

Now we average the two scores, 4.0 for technique and 3.5 for style, giving her a final score of 3.75 for the hail. You ain't gonna win no gold medal with that kind of number, lady.

I consider myself a liberal judge, perhaps giving away points too freely. I have awarded quite a few 5.9s that probably should have received a lower score, usually because I found myself enchanted by the style. In fact, I've always been a sucker for any of the *Specialty Hails:*

1. *The Nose Hail* – that's when the prospective passenger has both arms occupied and must therefore hail you with her nose. You

see a few of those every year around Christmas time.

2. *The Behind-the-Back Hail* – usually attempted from the sidewalk, this tricky hail is employed when two people are engrossed in conversation and the one doing the hailing doesn't want to interrupt what he's saying by turning and facing the oncoming cab. So he waves a hand behind his back to signal to the cab to stop *without actually looking at the cab.* When executed properly it is a thing of beauty.

3. *The Kissing Hail* – the same thing as the Behind-the-Back Hail except it's done while two people are engaged in the middle of a passionate kiss and one of them has to make a train.

4. *The Lasso Hail* (*'Laredo'*) – you see this hail occasionally from veteran New Yorkers who are standing at an intersection, see a cab approaching, raise their hand high in the air, make eye contact with the driver, and then communicate to the driver that they want him to turn into the intersection by about-facing and walking to the exact spot where they want the cabbie to stop, all the while keeping their hand up in the air. It's as if they had lassoed the taxi and were pulling it to its destination.

5. *The Window Hail* – usually seen during the evening rush hours, it's when a would-be passenger sees an unmoving cab on the street from inside a store or restaurant and hails the driver from behind the glass. The cabbie then pulls over and waits for his new passenger's arrival.

6. *The Tit Hail* (women only) – yes, I've seen it once. It was a Saturday night at 5 a.m. and the post-clubbing rush hour was

in full swing, making it impossible to get a cab for a while. A young lady, who no doubt had been drinking, flipped out a tit and was waving it at me as I approached her on Hudson Street in Greenwich Village. Most unfortunately, it was the end of my shift and I had to get the cab back to the garage, so I was off-duty and didn't pick her up – one of my life's great regrets.

7. *The Pissing Hail* (men only) – another one I've seen only once. A young rogue, drunk (of course), was pissing onto a mailbox on West 49th at 4 a.m. and hailed me in mid-pee as I came rolling down the street. 'Genius,' I thought, and I gave him a 5.9 on sheer originality alone.

But what about a 6.0, you may be wondering. What makes a hail a *perfect* hail? Besides being technically flawless, it has to be so brilliant, so never-seen-that-before, so charming, and at the same time so effortless, that it leaves you in awe. In all my years, I have awarded the coveted 6.0 only three times.

Whistled down

There are different kinds of whistles that people whistle. There's the 'here, boy' dog whistle. There's the macho mating call whistle when caveman sees girl. There are whistles for hot dog vendors at baseball games. And there are taxicab-hailing whistles.

It has its own distinct sound. When done correctly the taxi driver knows on hearing it that it's meant for him and him only. That's how it was one sunny day on Houston Street between Greene and Mercer in Soho.

I was cruising along on Houston at about thirty miles per hour, looking for my next fare, with the windows rolled down due to the pleasant weather. I drove past West Broadway, past Wooster, past Greene, and got almost to the corner of Mercer when it hit me square in the head like a heat-seeking dart.

The whistle came from the distant right-rear and I knew immediately that it was for me. There was no need to even check the rearview mirror. I just pulled over to the curb and stopped, then turned around to see who this marksman was. To my amazement, he was all the way back at Greene Street, nearly a full block away, an incredible distance from which to attempt the whistle hail. He was a middle-aged man with gray hair and beard, a bit overweight, dressed casually but smartly. He jogged without effort to the cab and smiled just enough to show that he was aware of the skill of his hail and was pleased to have accomplished it.

As he got in he thanked me for stopping, gave me his destination, and we were off. Through conversation I learned that he was an artist's rep and was coming from a gallery in Soho. It made sense that he was in the arts.

I reviewed the hail in my mind and could find nothing wrong. His style had an airy aesthetic to it and his technique… well, he had accomplished something that you would have thought was acoustically impossible and he did it with a smile.

A tour de force. A 6.0.

Long distance calling

Although it is no longer there, there was once a heliport on East 60th Street, bound by the East River on one side and York Avenue on the other. This heliport was atop a small hill, so if you were departing from it you would have to walk down this hill to get to York. Conversely, if you were coming toward the heliport from the opposite direction on 60th Street, you would also find yourself going down a small hill to get to York. So York at this particular intersection is like a little valley surrounded on both sides by higher elevations.

And that's where I was one October afternoon in 1985, waiting behind six or seven other cars for the light to turn green on 60th where it feeds into York. My roof light was on, indicating there were no passengers in the cab. From my position behind the steering wheel I could see all the way across York and onto the hill that leads to the heliport, a distance of about one city block.

I was looking out at that hill while waiting for the light to change when a man of about forty appeared there. Wearing a business suit and overcoat and carrying an attaché case in his right hand, he was obviously coming from the heliport. I suspected from the way he was walking, even at such a distance, that he was very possibly looking for a cab. He had that 'I want a cab' demeanor.

We were both at about the same elevation, enabling us potentially to make eye contact above the roofs of the cars in front of me. Sure enough, after glancing around for a moment and noticing me, his left hand went up *and pointed* to his left, indicating he wanted me to turn right on York. A few seconds later the light turned green and the traffic in front of me started moving slowly through the intersection. By the time I turned right on York, he was standing there waiting for me, having already crossed the avenue on foot.

He entered the cab, told me his destination, sat back, opened up the *Wall Street Journal*, and, with no mention of the remarkable cycle of communication that had just transpired, we proceeded to his apartment house on East 57th Street.

In terms of technique, obviously the hail was flawless – a full block away and he's able to tell me in which direction I should turn. As for style, I guess it was like listening to Pavarotti if you're an opera aficionado. A hail utterly fitting to someone whose self-confidence is on the brink of overflowing into smugness. A masterpiece, *a piéce de résistance.* A 6.0.

Bravo, maestro!

The sunroof hail

I had taken my last fare for the night, or at least I thought I had, and was heading east on 59th Street in the direction of the 59th Street Bridge – home to Queens. It happens once in a while that you can catch a late-night fare out to Queens on 59th Street, so I'm always extra alert for a sudden hail when I'm driving on this street after midnight.

I crossed Madison Avenue and was heading toward Park at about twenty-five miles per hour when a small car parked on the right side of the street caught my attention. There were three or four people in the car and the person sitting in the driver's seat seemed to be looking into his rearview mirror. I thought that was odd and kept looking over at the vehicle as I approached it. Suddenly a hand shot up through the car's sunroof and waved back and forth. I instinctively moved my eyes to the hand and then back to the rearview mirror and saw two eyes, eyebrows raised, staring at me. I understood the communication – I was being hailed! I pulled the cab over to the left side of the street and stopped.

Two young ladies in party dresses emerged from the car, blew kisses at the driver, crossed the street, and got into my cab. The driver, who appeared to be what might be called a 'cool dude', smiled broadly at them, blew kisses back, and drove off straight down 59th Street toward the bridge. The girls wanted to go uptown, but their friend was heading out to Queens himself and was in too much of a rush, apparently, to make a detour, so they'd decided to take a cab. I made a left on Park and we scooted up to 93rd Street, where they got out.

It took me a minute or two to really comprehend what I'd just seen. This guy had made eye contact with me, backwards through a mirror, while I was in motion. He'd hailed me, also backwards, by shooting his arm up through the roof of a car. And he'd done it so well that it worked. And to put a cherry on it, he didn't seem to think, from his demeanor, that he'd done anything special. Perfectly in character for a 'cool dude'. To say it was a 6.0 would be an understatement. It may have been the greatest hail in the history of hails!

Now, what we've seen with these stories of 6.0s is the top of the line when it comes to obtaining the services of a taxi in New York City. But there is an underbelly here, too, which can suddenly become visible when demand exceeds supply. Let's say you've been trying to get a cab for twenty minutes in a cold rain on a Midtown street and are surrounded on all sides by other people, now your competitors, in the same situation. A cab stops to let a passenger out but some son of a bitch, or the bitch herself, grabs it first, a cab that should have been *yours.* As minutes continue to tick by and you're becoming late for your appointment, you feel the thin veneer of civilization beginning to strip away. A subway is no longer an option. You need a cab *now!*

You have entered a little zone of human conduct where the expected niceties suddenly do not apply. In fact, it's an area where you can see what people are really made of because there are no consequences for bad behavior. Hustle your way in front of some sucker who was about to get into a cab? Why not? You'll never see him again and even if you did, he wouldn't remember you, anyway.

Most of these incidents, ugly as they may be, end right there. Rightfully or wrongfully, one person gets the cab and the other is left in the lurch. If I see two people hailing me in the same spot, I try to stop the cab in the middle of them so I'm not appearing to take sides. Then I let them work it out (or slug it out) between themselves. But sometimes neither contestant will back down and the cabbie inevitably becomes the arbiter of the dispute, sort of an impromptu referee.

Wisdom

I was cruising down Broadway on a brutally cold January evening at the height of the rush hour when I spotted several desperate-looking people waving in my direction from the far side of 14th Street. I brought the cab to a stop without choosing a favorite and waited to see who would wind up in possession of my precious, yellow object. Two twenty-something males simultaneously got in from opposite sides of the cab and sat down, neither acknowledging the presence of the other. Both told me his destination – one uptown and one downtown, so there could be no sharing – and ignored the other. There was no discussion between them as to who had the cab first. It was simply up to me.

I turned around and looked at them. I could tell by the expressions on their faces that neither was going to back down and the situation had the potential of getting nasty. It was as if they were both fastened to the seat by an imaginary chain. What to do?

Now, if I may digress for moment, disputes over possession of cabs can be broken down by gender. If it's man versus woman, the woman usually wins. Most men, even in this age, have an innate sense of chivalry when it comes to physical matters with the opposite sex. Women, knowing this, sometimes use it to their advantage. I have occasionally overheard two girls giggling to each other, after being given possession of my taxi by some guy who clearly had it first, as if to say, 'Thanks, sucker'. If it's woman versus woman, however, watch out. I have heard some very unladylike language and even seen some shoving to gain an advantage. But that's about as far as it would ever go. I think women know that in a confrontation with another woman the worst case scenario might involve some hair-pulling or kicking, but that's it. Man versus man, however, is another matter, and that's because men know on a gut level that a real fight with another man can mean serious injury or even death. Or jail. So men tend to not let things go too far before one of them, sensibly, backs down.

But these guys had taken it a step too far. One of them was going to lose not only a cab, but face. And I wasn't sure there wouldn't be violence right there in my cab. *What to do?*

The solution suddenly came to me in a flash, giving me the thought that perhaps I'd missed out on what could have been a fulfilling career in the diplomatic corps. All that was needed was the same procedure that has resolved conflicts since the Stone Age – *the coin toss.*

After getting their agreement, I pulled out a quarter. Downtown said 'heads', Uptown said 'tails', and the coin went flipping up into the air. 'Tails' it was and Downtown exited with no dispute and a full face.

Hey, they don't call me 'Salomon' for nuthin'.

After the opera

Oddly enough, the most vile, sneaky, down-and-dirty, knife-in-the-back fights for empty cabs take place at Lincoln Center just after the opera, ballet or symphony have let out. In fact, watching the highbrows maneuver around each other in their attempts to snatch up available taxis before anyone else can get them might be considered more entertaining by some than the performance they had just attended.

I had been cruising up Amsterdam Avenue on a Saturday night at about 10.30 p.m., looking for my next fare, when I made a right on 65th Street, the northern border of Lincoln Center. Realizing the shows would soon be ending and there would be tons of people wanting rides, I thought I would sit in the taxi stand on Columbus Avenue for a few minutes until the first ones came running out. But before I could cross all the way to Columbus, a woman darted out of a side entrance on 65th Street, eagerly waving her hand in the classic 'I want a taxi' manner.

She appeared to be about sixty-five years old and was dressed in a red evening gown. I pulled over to the curb and stopped. As she opened the back door and started to get in, I noticed that a man who'd been standing on the sidewalk about thirty yards further down the street had started to run toward me at a full gallop. He was around forty-five years old, bald, and was dressed in a black tuxedo.

The woman had closed her door and was telling me her destination as the man came hustling up. Normally I would have driven away as soon as the back door had been closed, but, with the man running toward us the way he was, I thought the two of them might have been together, so I just waited there a moment until he arrived.

He opened the back door.

'Excuse *me*,' he said to my passenger, 'but apparently you did not bother to notice that I'd been standing there hailing this cab before you took it for yourself. This is *my* cab. Please get out.'

'I *beg* your pardon?' she replied, shocked and confused.

'Get out of the cab. This is *my* cab.'

'I will *not*!'

'Madam,' he said, 'do you want me to *drag* you out of the taxi? It may come as a surprise to you to know that there are people in this world who are not willing to let others walk all over them, even by elderly women such as yourself.'

'I *beg* your pardon!'

Apparently the man in the tuxedo had done enough talking and, being a man of action, he went to work at showing my passenger that he meant every word he'd said – he grabbed her by the arm and started pulling her out of the cab!

'Get your hands off of me!' she screamed, and she latched onto the headrest on top of the front seat with her free hand to prevent herself from being literally dragged out to the street.

At this point I realized that taxi driver intervention was urgently needed, so I turned around and spoke sharply to the lunatic in the tux.

'Listen, pal,' I said, 'even if you manage to pull her out of my cab, I'm not driving you anywhere. So you might as well just let her go.'

He looked at me with an expression of hurt surprise – as if some unspoken bond between us had been broken – released the woman's arm, and stepped back from the cab. She immediately slammed her door shut, but I wasn't done giving him a piece of my mind, so I leaned over and yelled at him through the open window.

'Is this how you prove to yourself how tough you are? By dragging old ladies out of taxis? You goddamned idiot!' And with that I stepped on the gas and wheeled on out of there toward Columbus, thinking it would be great if my spinning wheels could spread some righteous dust all over the guy.

'Where would you like to go, ma'am?' I asked her gently.

'81st and West End,' she said rather coldly.

I made a left on Broadway and headed in that direction. I thought what I'd done was brilliantly effective and really quite nice as far as my passenger was concerned and I was hoping a 'thank you' or some sign of appreciation would be forthcoming, so I tried to engage her in conversation about her little ordeal.

'I can't believe what that nut was trying to do to you,' I said. 'My God, talk about chivalry being dead!'

But my comment was met with a stony silence. I tried again.

'What a pathetic human being that guy was,' I said.

Again my words hit a brick wall. I looked at her through the mirror and saw that she was staring rather blankly out of her window, apparently immersed in her own thoughts and oblivious to whatever I might have to say. So I decided to just let her be and not talk any further unless she spoke to me. She was probably too shook up to feel comfortable talking to a stranger about it.

It took five minutes of silent driving to get her up to 81st Street. The fare was $3.25. She handed me three singles and two quarters, a particularly tiny tip, especially considering how I'd rescued her. She started to depart, stepping out onto the street, but before she closed her door she finally spoke.

'Thank you for your help,' she said, 'but I want you to know that I do *not* consider myself to be an *old lady!*'

And with that she closed her door rather sharply and walked off in what might have been a huff toward her apartment building.

Oh.

You know, I don't consider myself to be a particularly timid individual, but I've got to tell you I don't cruise the streets around Lincoln Center too much anymore. I've added it to a list that includes the South Bronx, the Port Authority Bus Terminal and leather bars as places that are too risky to one's health to get too close to.

I mean, this job is dangerous enough – why take crazy chances?

17

At Journey's End

There are two basic dynamics at play in the game of taxi driving in New York City. The first is what goes on when there's a passenger in the cab – you have the goal of getting to a specific Point B and along with that there's the interplay, or lack of interplay, between yourself and the passenger. And the second begins at journey's end, when you are once again alone and looking for that next traveling companion.

If you drive the night shift (5 p.m. to 5 a.m.) as I do, there are plenty of traveling companions up until midnight. After that hour, however, with the exception of Fridays and Saturdays, it's as if someone has turned off the faucet. Passengers become scarcer and scarcer as the night wears on and a rather ferocious competition for finding them takes place among the drivers. When it gets beyond 2 a.m., it's not uncommon to go half an hour or more between fares.

Many drivers, myself included, have developed their own personal 'cruising routes' as a solution to this problem. Experience teaches us that certain parts of town, certain streets, even certain *sides* of these certain streets, are the most optimum for finding the next passenger at certain times of the night. These cruising routes are closely guarded secrets. No cabbie tells another what they are for fear the word would get out and his little treasure chest would be looted. If, however, you should ask me what *my* cruising routes are, I'll be glad to tell you. Just be aware that I'll be lying.

But there are times during these late-night hours when I become weary of the endless racing with my fellow drivers in order to maintain 'position' on the avenues. I fall away from the pack and just start to wander, with no particular strategy in mind. It's at these times, perhaps just out of sheer loneliness, that the city itself becomes my companion. My thoughts turn to this intriguing creation and once again I find myself on its wavelength, a true believer, cruising along, hoping that a further insight into what it, and therefore what it all, is all about will somehow find its way into my taxi and land on my shoulder.

Ah, New York! Like a great character in a great story, the contradictions in its personality keep you fascinated by it. Its qualities are so inspiring, its underbelly so disturbing, its mood swings so sudden and its significance so enormous that many of the brightest and most adventurous among us feel its gravitational pull: a continuing urge to approach it, to get into it, to be a part of it, to ride its waves and, internalizing its challenges, to master it.

Many years ago a passenger shared with me what I thought was a particularly astute insight about New York. Throughout history, he said, every empire has had its principal city, its central location where its business is conducted and its culture propagated. During the Roman Empire, it was Rome. During the British Empire, London. Although in today's world, with our high-speed communication and transportation abilities, the point where an empire begins and ends may not be as clear as it once was, I still think there's a lot of truth in that observation. More than any other location, New York City is the center of today's world. And that is the source of the 'energy' so many people say they perceive when they come here, an energy they feel does not exist anywhere else. 'There is no other place like it' is a comment I hear quite often from world travelers.

So come with me now at journey's end for a final ride around this town. Let us wander, ghost-like, in and out of its darkened passageways. Let me show you what New York City is, what it was, and perhaps what it could be, at least according to me.

Jump in.

Uh, sorry, I don't think your door is closed all the way.

Thank you.

Okay, we're off. Let's go all the way down to the southern tip of Manhattan Island, where it all began with the first Dutch settlers back in 1624. Stopping at Rector and Broadway, we can see Trinity Church and its ancient (by American standards) cemetery, one of the very few still remaining in Manhattan. Look through the iron fence. There is the oblong-shaped gravestone of Alexander Hamilton, whose picture is on the ten-dollar bill. More than any of the founding fathers, it is in Hamilton's vision of America, it has been said, that we live today. And yet his modest stone is not even the largest in the cemetery. That in itself speaks volumes about America.

Just a block away is Wall Street, today so heavily guarded you'd think you were in a war zone. Did you know that New York was the first capital of the United States? Look down the street. There's Federal Hall, the exact spot where George Washington took the oath of office as the first president of this country on April 30, 1789. Circling around a few blocks uptown, there is St Paul's Chapel, the oldest standing church in New York. Inside that church is the pew where Washington prayed, and hanging above it is the original painting of the Great Seal of the United States, which you see depicted on the back of the one-dollar bill. A passenger once told me it had been her job in the bicentennial year of 1976 to escort that iconic image to a ceremony in Philadelphia and that she had received a police escort from the airport to the place where the event took place. I always remember that story when I'm stuck in traffic and some motorcade zips by – I could be granting right-of-way to a painting!

Okay, we make a right on Fulton and go one block down the street to Church. Yes, there it is – the place that was once so sadly known as 'Ground Zero'.

It will probably always be impossible to drive by this area without thinking about what happened. I have been asked many times by tourists in my cab where I was on that day, and I have two answers to that question: first, that I was there at the World Trade Center on September 11; and second, that I was home sleeping on September 11. Both are true statements. You see, I drove the night shift on September 10. At around 2 a.m., then September 11, I took a woman from Greenwich Village to the PATH station (the subway that goes to New Jersey) at the foot of the North Tower. When the shift was over at 5 a.m., I went home to sleep. Waking at noon, and then preparing for just another work day, I was informed of the disaster by my daughter. The concept that, merely eight hours after I had dropped that woman off, the World Trade Center would cease to exist still seems surreal to me. Anyone who had ever stood directly beneath the towers and seen with his own eyes their utter immensity will understand the impossibility of this happening. And yet, of course, it did.

The days, weeks and months that followed are set aside in a sacred time capsule in my mind. The great majority of New Yorkers had never suffered a disaster firsthand. Massive calamities were things we'd heard about in the news all our lives, but here? Never. Our former misfortunes had generally been experienced on a personal basis, but this was something that happened to *us*.

And the 'us' of New York City emerged as it never had before in our lifetimes. The undercurrent of community which had often been barely perceptible in the Monster City became a river of caring and helping. Patriotism, a sentiment considered by many to be beneath their level of sophistication, came out of the closet. For the first time in my life I decided to display an American flag, and it appeared on the rear window of my taxi.

Riding around the city in those first days, the things that most jolted you were the physical results of the attack. There was the shock of seeing the skyline for the first time without the buildings, their dominance replaced by an unending tower of smoke. There was the smell, an odd and disturbing stench that could not be identified as anything you'd ever encountered before. There were the restrictions on traveling downtown. There was the presence of military and emergency units everywhere. And there was an eerie emptiness both of vehicles and people in Times Square, its bright lights still shining but seeming now so strangely inappropriate.

And then the posters began appearing – first a few, then a torrent, going up on walls, on lampposts and in storefront windows: 'MISSING' (a name and a picture), 'LAST SEEN ON THE 104TH FLOOR' (the name of the company the person worked for) and 'PLEASE CALL (a number) IF YOU HAVE ANY INFORMATION'. On the evening of September 13, as I emerged from a Starbucks with a cup of coffee in my hand, I saw a young woman take such a poster from a stack she was carrying and hurriedly tape it onto a mailbox. The look of grim determination on her face, the speed with which she worked, and then her marching off to find the next place to attach one told me something of what so many people were going through. These were the friends and relatives who had waited in desperation for a telephone call that never came.

As time went on, New Yorkers became each other's therapists. When a passenger arrived in my cab, I would begin the ride by asking, 'How are you doing?', not so much as a way of saying hello, but because I really wanted to know how they were doing and to help them by listening. And they often did the same for me. Gradually the need to talk about the tragedy began to lessen, and after about a year our period of mutual mourning was coming to an end. The city was becoming its 'old self' once again. And what is that old self? We'll get to that in a minute, but first, hey, look out the window, I want to show you something.

Have you noticed that as we are traveling uptown in Manhattan that when we get to a certain point (Houston Street) in the lower part of the island the streets no longer have names? We are entering 'the grid' – straight streets and straight avenues, all intersecting at perpendicular angles, all pretty much the same distance from each other, and all – well, nearly all – having numbers instead of names. It makes Manhattan a very easy place in which to get around. Now, for a taxi driver this is obviously a big deal, as the majority of his rides will be within the grid. But it turns out the construction of the grid is part of the answer to an important history lesson that explains how New York became the Monster City of the World and helps us understand what it is today.

Let's take, by comparison, Boston, Philadelphia and Baltimore – three major cities with basically the same early history as New York. All were founded as English colonies in the 1600s and all are on the Atlantic Ocean, only a few hundred miles from each other. And yet, a few centuries later, New York has more than three times the population of these other three cities *combined.*

Why?

It's actually because of a canal. No, not the little one that once ran across lower Manhattan and for which Canal Street is named – the *big one*, the Erie Canal that connected two upstate cities, Albany and Buffalo. Here's the story…

In the year 1811 the governor of New York State, DeWitt Clinton, took a look at a map. There was New York City at the mouth of the Hudson River. If you went up the river 153 miles, there was Albany, the capital of the state. If you then looked westward on the map, there was Buffalo, three hundred miles from Albany. Just a small town at the time, Buffalo was located on Lake Erie, one of the five Great Lakes. These Great Lakes are all connected to each other and extend westward halfway across the continent, all the way to Minnesota, a distance from Buffalo of about a thousand miles.

This meant that when the construction of the Erie Canal was completed, materials could travel from the harbor of New York City all the way across the wide-open country by water, which at the time was enormously cheaper, faster and easier than trying to ship them by land. Remember, there were few or no trains back then and the roads that existed were completely inadequate to handle the settlement of the frontier.

The significance of this cannot be overstated. It meant you could now get building materials quickly, safely and inexpensively to the newly settled territories. You could ship a piano to Ohio. It meant that what it would take to create America, this incredible explosion of commerce, was all going to begin in New York City.

Realizing this, the government of New York began the construction of the street grid of Manhattan at the same time as the Erie Canal. So when the canal was opened for business in 1825, the infrastructure needed to handle the commerce it would generate was already in place. Talk about 'build it and they will come'!

And come they did. They came from all over the world, they came quickly, and they came in vast numbers. By the year 1900 the city's population had grown to twenty times what it had been in 1825 – over three million people of differing languages, races and religions all jammed together on a small island. It was the greatest social experiment in the history of the human race.

Riding through the Lower East Side so late at night, we can almost see them looking out at us there on Hester Street, on Delancey, on Rivington, on Essex. The Irish, the Italians, the Russians, the Chinese, the Germans, the Jews, and a bit of everyone else – this is where their voyages as immigrants ended and their new lives as Americans began.

This multi-cultural rubbing together of shoulders continues to this day and has resulted in the values and characteristics that are typical of a New Yorker. Actually, it has resulted in *this story…*

Nonchalance

> Nonchalance: the state of being characterized by or showing a lack of interest or enthusiasm; casually indifferent. (*Macmillan Dictionary for Students*)

In New York City nonchalance is something that is earned by years of residing there. It comes from being bombarded by so many offbeat and unexpected realities that one finally develops a tolerance to them. Not a pretended tolerance, but a true tolerance. In fact, the determination of who's a 'real' New Yorker and who is not could probably be best made by measuring a person's level of nonchalance.

I had a fare on a Wednesday afternoon in December, 1984 which introduced me to a person who had earned an advanced degree in this characteristic. I had pulled over in a bus stop on Columbus Avenue at 62nd Street, right in front of Lincoln Center, due to a minor emergency in the middle of the work day – my meter had run out of receipt paper and, since the damned things won't work at all if they run out of paper, I had to attend to it immediately.

I was busy trying to place the paper into the feed when the right rear door suddenly opened and an unexpected customer entered my cab.

It was a clown.

Not a figurative clown, a *real* clown, in a polka dot suit with a funny hat, a painted face and a bright red nose. I had forgotten to put on my off-duty light and had left the doors unlocked, so he understandably figured I was working.

'57th and Broadway, please,' he said matter-of-factly, not acknowledging by his words or demeanor that there was anything out of the ordinary about his appearance. It was a demonstration of some gutsy nonchalance.

'Could you wait a second until I get this paper in the meter?' I asked, not showing any particular surprise or special interest in the fact that here I was, out of nowhere, suddenly conversing with a full-fledged clown. (I'm not too low on the scale of nonchalance myself, if you don't mind my saying so.)

'Okay,' he said, 'I'm just trying to get to the bank before it closes at three.'

The clock on my taxi's dashboard showed that it was ten minutes before the hour.

'I'll get you there with time to spare,' I said, and within a few seconds I had the paper in the meter and we were on our way. His destination was only a minute's drive from where we were starting, so arriving there before closing time would be no problem.

I realized as we pulled out into the traffic on Columbus that he must be from the Big Apple Circus which was in town at the time and performing in a tent in a park that's just behind Lincoln Center. He was probably on a break between shows.

'Gotta make a deposit before closing,' he said as we made a left on 57th Street, 'or I'm gonna bounce a check.'

I wondered what a personal check from a clown might look

like – would it have a picture of balloons and elephants on it? – but I didn't say anything. It wouldn't have been nonchalant to have brought it up.

'Don't worry, buddy, you're as good as there,' I said, and in fact we did arrive within a minute. I pulled over into an open area right next to the curb and waited for him to pay me. But instead of money I received a request.

'Would you mind waiting for me while I'm in the bank,' he asked, 'and then take me back to where you picked me up? I'll give you a good tip.'

'No problem,' I replied, and I left the clock running. He jumped out of the cab and hurried into the bank.

It took him longer in there than I'd expected. I could see him in the bank from where I was parked, and I noticed that he was waiting in a line – a single file consisting of two young women, an elderly man and a clown – and I guessed there must have been only one or two tellers on duty. Eventually I began to daydream a bit and I found myself wondering how many clowns could fit into my cab. Wouldn't it be something, I thought, if I pulled into the driveway of a big hotel, the doorman opens the rear door, and a stream of twenty clowns comes pouring out, each one dressed more colorfully than the one before him? Or how about thirty clowns? Or maybe if…

My reverie was broken by his reappearance.

'Thanks,' he said as he jumped back in the cab, 'now could you just drop me back on 62nd Street, please.'

'Will do,' I said, and I steered the cab back out into the moving lanes of 57th Street, made a couple of turns, and headed back uptown. I was curious to know more about his big emergency, so I inquired about it.

'What was in danger of bouncing, your rent check?' I asked.

'No,' he replied, 'I'm a student of American history and a few days ago I secured an autograph of Aaron Burr with a postdated check. I had to make sure *that* check didn't bounce.'

I thought this was quite interesting and asked him a couple of questions about the value of autographs of figures in American history and what his collection consisted of, and we were becoming involved in a lively discussion on the subject when we arrived back at 62nd and Columbus. The meter was up to five-fifty. He handed me eight dollars, told me to keep it, and left the cab, heading down 62nd in the direction of the Big Apple Circus.

As I filled in my trip sheet, I noted mentally that I had never acknowledged that he was dressed as a clown, he had never acknowledged that he was dressed as a clown, and none of the passersby on the street, either in front of the bank or at Columbus Avenue, had stared at him, smiled at him, or in any way paid any special attention to him.

It was New York City at its pinnacle of magnificence.

Chalance

All right, now we know what nonchalance is and we know that it is a characteristic of a 'real' New Yorker. But how about a word to describe someone who's *not* a 'real' New Yorker – a fraud? New York, the city with everything, has plenty of those, too. This word should be the opposite of 'nonchalance' and it should be, of course, 'chalance'. But after having searched through every dictionary from Webster to Schmebster, I have concluded that, due to some quirk of etymology, the word 'chalance' does not exist.

Well, it does now. I'm inventing it right here and I'm defining it as 'the state or condition of showing excitement, surprise, or dismay at things that are out of the ordinary'. It could also be defined as 'pretended nonchalance'. 'Chalant', to make it an adjective, would be how I would describe a passenger in my cab who had to be the complete opposite of the clown from the Big Apple Circus.

I didn't know his name, but to me he was 'Joe Cool'. He was a young, good-looking guy who got in my cab at 3rd Avenue and 25th Street with two young, good-looking girls on a rainy night in September, 1985. He wasted no time in going into his

Joe Cool persona.

'Eugene, my man,' he brayed after checking out my name on my hack license, 'have I got a great fare for you, or what?'

I was instantly on guard. This guy was trying to sell me something and that sets the alarm bells ringing.

'To Brooklyn, Ocean Parkway and Avenue P,' he continued, 'and then – now listen to this, Eugene, because I know you cab drivers all hate to go to Brooklyn – and then you take me back right here! And I'm payin' you twenty up front so you won't think I'm tryin' to rip you off.' And with that he handed me a twenty. All before I could say hello.

I looked at the bill. It seemed fine.

'All right,' I said, 'let's go.' I made a couple of turns and headed for the FDR Drive. We were on our way.

I hated to admit it to myself, but he was right. I usually *do* hate to go to Brooklyn and if a passenger tells me he wants to take a very long and unusual ride, I *am* thinking it might be the start of some kind of rip-off. But he was paying me up front. I had nothing to object to.

'What are you doing, picking someone up in Brooklyn?' I asked as we entered the rain-soaked highway.

'See these two gorgeous chicks?' Joe Cool replied, 'these are the hottest, most beautiful babes in all of New York City. I'm taking them home, that's all.'

Looking in the rearview mirror, I could see that he was sitting between the girls and had an arm around each of them. One leaned her head against his shoulder and the other used her free hand to play with his hair. It was a picture made in macho heaven with an underlying tint of hefty nonchalance, but somehow the thing wasn't ringing true. My sixth sense was telling me that I wasn't looking at real nonchalance here. What I was seeing was… well, I didn't want to be overly judgmental on the guy. After all, he had paid me up front.

After ten minutes of sluggish driving on the FDR, we arrived at the ramp leading onto the Brooklyn Bridge. The traffic was slower than usual due to the rain and my attention had been drawn primarily to controlling the motion of the cab on the slippery pavement. There was a continual flow of chatter, flirting and silly laughter coming from the back seat to which I had become accustomed and figured would be with me until the girls had been dropped off in Brooklyn, so I was surprised when Joe suddenly broke the pattern and asked me to turn my radio onto a hard rock station.

I moved the dial until I found a station he liked. As the harsh sound came blaring out of the speakers, I glanced in the mirror and saw that Joe and the girls had transformed themselves into rock singers. Joe had put on a pair of sunglasses and was sitting up in his seat mouthing the words of the song on the radio. The girls were his backup group and were making sensual motions with their bodies as they lip-synched along with Joe.

'Eugene,' Joe called out, taking a quick break from his set, 'turn it up, dude.'

I figured what the hell and complied. Sure, he was a bona fide jerk, but he'd only be in my life for another thirty minutes, so why make waves? I kept my eyes on the road.

It took another ten minutes to get them to their destination on Ocean Parkway, ten minutes of remarkable tolerance on my part considering how annoying my passengers had become and that their money was already in my pocket. But, anyway, we were there. Joe ran out with the girls to the entrance of the apartment building, kissed them both passionately, and then hustled back to my cab, taking off his sunglasses as he jumped in. As we began our drive back to Manhattan, I noticed a change in his personality.

'Do you mind if I smoke a cigarette?' he asked politely.

I told him I had no problem with that and he lit up, opening his window a little to help with the ventilation. I noticed that he kept his cigarettes in an elegant gold box, a touch of refinement. He sat back and extended his arms across the top of his seat and appeared to be in complete comfort, as if he were relaxing in his favorite chair in his own living room. He drew deeply on his Marlboro.

'How about if we switch to a jazz station?' he asked. 'Would that be all right with you?'

Jazz would be a welcome change from hard rock, so I gladly started to flip through the dial. Suddenly I realized how Joe had changed. He was still Joe Cool, but it was a variation on the theme. It had gone from a Fonzie kind of cool to a Lou Rawls kind of cool. More mellow and mature, can you dig?

We moved along cautiously on Ocean Parkway which, although called a parkway, is actually a wide, residential road. It ends by leading into the Prospect Expressway, which really is a highway. As we entered the Prospect, the rain started coming down even harder and I adjusted my driving style into full-alert mode, which means two hands on the wheel, wipers on high, a slower speed, and plenty of room between the cab and the other vehicles on the road. Joe, however, was oblivious to the weather. He had something to say.

'I prefer women who've reached a plateau of self-realization regarding their own sexuality,' he proclaimed. 'Women who understand that to be fulfilled means never having enough. Women who are into the creation of joy.'

'Oh.'

'Lisa and Gabrielle back there?'

'Yeah?'

'We just made love for two hours. The three of us. Have you

ever experienced that kind of heaven, man?'

'Well, I'm married, you know, and I, uh, well, you know…'

I was struggling for a way to say "no" and still retain my masculinity on an equal footing with his own when I realized that he didn't care what I said, anyway. Joe Cool was the Master of Love and this was a time for contented reflection. I shut up.

'Heaven. Heaven. Just the joy of heaven, do you understand?'

I was wondering why, if there was a God, He was making me listen to this when we were suddenly confronted with a serious emergency on the road. A car ahead of us had hydroplaned out of control and crashed into a retaining wall on our right and the car directly in front of us was spinning completely around and showing us, instead of its taillights, its headlights. It was a situation in which, as a driver, you must act expertly and instantly in order to avoid becoming part of an accident. My job was made more difficult by one additional factor: Joe Cool was freaking out.

'WHOA! WHOA! OKAY! WHOA!' he screamed as he lunged forward and clutched onto both of my shoulders for support. 'WHOA! WHOA! WATCHIT! WHOA!'

I pumped the brakes gently and kept my eyes firmly on the car in front of us. Joe continued to grasp me desperately from behind and attempted to steer the cab by exerting pressure on my shoulders, first to the left and then to the right.

'IT'S OKAY! IT'S OKAY! WE'RE GONNA BE OKAY!' he screamed in unmitigated terror.

I ignored him and continued to pump the brakes. When my cab had slowed down sufficiently, I checked that no other vehicles were approaching from behind us, pulled out carefully into the lane on our left, and passed the turned-around car without going into a spin of our own. If I don't say so myself, it was damned good driving. Joe seemed satisfied that the danger had passed and released his grip on my shoulders.

'You all right, man?' I asked.

'It's okay, it's okay,' he said, more to himself than to me. Then he sat back in his seat, apparently drained of all emotion and perhaps in some kind of state of shock.

It took me another fifteen minutes or so to get him back to 3rd Avenue and 25th Street. Except for saying goodbye at the end of the ride, we didn't have any further conversation. The meter went up to eighteen dollars and change and the amount left over from the twenty was my tip.

They say you can tell what people are made of in times of emergency. Do they show grace under pressure, a firm resolve, a steadiness that inspires confidence? Do they exhibit the kind of hard-edged determination that makes you feel these are the kinds of people you'd like to have around when the going gets tough?

Or do they show something else – something not quite so inspiring, something that makes you think that maybe you'd be better off if they weren't there at all?

Do they show – what was that word?

Oh, yes.

Chalance.

Ah, Joe Cool. Riding around the city in these empty hours before dawn, I see him still in my mind's eye as I zip uptown on 3rd Avenue in the Gramercy section of town. I still see the llama on Central Park South – where did he bring that llama at the end of the night, anyway? – and I see Jackie Kennedy there, too. Cruising up into the Upper East Side, there's the building into which that pretty blonde disappeared, ripping me off for a ten-dollar fare. 'Pinky promise,' she said. And what about that guy who paid for the ride with a rib roast? Where could he be today? And the girl walking around with a pillow under her dress to trick people into thinking she was pregnant? What's become of her? She was smiling as she waved goodbye to me at Tompkins Square in the East Village…

…'I love you,' she said…

What a collection of characters you acquire when you drive a taxi in this city.

Now, look, here's something I want to show you at 96th and Park – it's a wall. Look, can you see it? No, you can't, because it's invisible, but it's as solid and forbidding in a social sense as the old Berlin Wall. Of all the dividing lines in New York which separate one type of people from another, there are none so distinct, none so black and white, as the difference between the north and south sides of 96th Street at Park Avenue. On the south, you have the American Aristocracy – prep schools, debutante balls and the Metropolitan Museum of Art. On the north, it's the barrio – bodegas, salsa music, and men in their undershirts playing dominoes on card tables on the sidewalks in the summer months. And although there are no cement blocks anywhere in sight, you might as well need a passport to get through it, for you never – *never!* – see anyone on either side of 96th who doesn't belong to his or her own side of the street.

The American Aristocracy – now there's an oxymoron for you. We're not supposed to have an aristocracy in the United States. When the American Revolution ended in 1783, the British and all their royalty and privileged nobility were shown the door. Instead, what was established was a level playing field based not on birth, but on ability. One man, one vote. A representative government. Equal justice for all. Surely there could be no aristocracy in

America.

But there is.

If you drive a cab in New York, you learn where they live. They live on Park and 5th Avenues between 60th and 96th Streets. If that's your address, good news, you are a member of the American upper class. And you're not merely 'well off', you're stinking rich, rolling in it, and most likely your parents, grandparents and great-grandparents were, too.

I actually look at the American Aristocracy as a kind of ethnic group that has its own particular characteristics in somewhat the same way that other such groups in the city do. There are sections of New York that are primarily identified by the places their residents originally came from or by the languages they speak: Spanish Harlem, Chinatown, Astoria with its Greeks, Flushing with its Koreans, and so on. And there are other sections of the city that are places most closely associated with people who have similar interests or lifestyles: disaffected, artistic twenty-somethings in the East Village, gays in Chelsea, aspiring actors in overpriced, four-story walk-ups in Hell's Kitchen.

Park Avenue and 5th Avenue between 60th and 96th are the places where you find people with the common denominators of having been born into or married into significant wealth, having never had to get a job to pay for their living expenses, and having the doors of opportunity always in the unlocked position. That's what you find in that part of town.

As a taxi driver, you have this fascinating vantage point from which to observe the characteristics of people from all these groups. I don't like to generalize, but as experience grows and one observes similar traits in certain types of people, some amount of generalization becomes inevitable. And here's what I have come to expect from members of the American Aristocracy:

a) polite children,

b) rowdy teenagers when in a group and not accompanied by an adult,

c) ten to fifteen percent tips – *never* excessive,

d) businesslike attitudes,

e) never drunk or loud,

f) non-conversational.

Now, none of these is too bad and polite children are good, but there is one other characteristic that I must say can really get under my skin. It's an attitude I sometimes pick up on that I am being considered a servant, a lesser-than, a non-person. It's not done blatantly, it's a nuance thing, but when I perceive it and then consider it's coming from someone who has never had to be concerned about how to pay the rent, it stirs up considerable resentment.

Riding with the American aristocracy

On a beautiful evening in July, 2007 I was hailed at the corner of 83rd Street and Madison Avenue by a waiter. He came up to the side of my cab and asked me to make a left on 83rd and pull up in front of his restaurant, Giovanni's, a little hole in the wall Italian joint I'd never noticed before. A regular customer would be coming out, he said – one who would tip me well, he assured me – and would I mind waiting a minute or two? Please?

Well, sure, I said, no problem, and then as he went back into the restaurant I started to contemplate how many times I'd been told how well I was going to be tipped only to find later that what I was given was at best an average gratuity. God, it happens all the time but, really, who cares? A good tip versus a lousy tip is a matter of a small amount of money, anyway, so why should he think this would be an inducement to me? Whatever…

It took a minute or so for the waiter to reappear and then I realized why there had been some anxiety in his manner. There wasn't one passenger, there were three – a man who looked to be about seventy years old, an elderly woman in a wheelchair, and a young, black woman whom I immediately understood to be her nurse. Some taxi drivers are cruelly unwilling to put up with the hassle of getting a wheelchair-bound passenger into the cab and have been known to drive off. I suspected that this may have happened to this waiter in the past, but he needn't have been concerned. I would never do that, of course.

I was ready to assist the crippled woman into the back seat and put the wheelchair into the trunk, but it turned out this was the job of the nurse. So all I had to do was watch the proceedings and say a few words to my passengers to make them feel at ease. I asked the elderly lady if she had enjoyed her meal, but instead of getting a response I got only a blank stare. Judging by her lack of reaction to anything that was going on around her, I realized she was in a demented state, or perhaps Alzheimer's or just 'senility' would be better words to describe her condition. In any case, this was a sad story I was witnessing.

When they were finally all in the cab, the gentleman, who sat in the front seat with me, told me that their destination was 75th Street and 5th Avenue, a very short ride to a prime American Aristocracy location. As we made the left from 83rd onto 5th it occurred to me that I have had far more elderly, wheelchair-bound passengers in my cab who were from Park or 5th Avenue buildings than I've had from other parts of the city. And I realized the reason for this was that wealthy people can afford to pay for the care of their elderly in their own homes. Others not so fortunate are placed in nursing homes or die at a younger age. It seemed to me to be yet another example of the privilege of the wealthy.

The ride down 5th Avenue to 75th Street was a silent one, the man sitting next to me saying not a word. When I stopped the cab in front of their building a doorman came running out to open the door and the procedure of extricating the elderly lady from the back seat went into motion with the nurse and the doorman doing the lifting. Finally, when the work was finished, the gentleman to my right reached into his pocket to pay me the $4.90 fare. I braced myself for a sixty-cent tip.

But I was wrong. He gave me a ten and told me to keep the change. Then he did something that was much more meaningful to me than an excellent tip. As we watched the elderly woman being wheeled into the building he looked at me with an expression on his face that conveyed the weight of the burden I suspected he'd been carrying for quite some time. And he spoke these words:

'Don't get old,' he said.

It said something to me I already knew but needed to be reminded of again – that if you've got enough food to eat and a roof over your head, you're living in the same neighborhood as the guy on 5th Avenue.

The human condition does not have a street address.

But it does have a city. I know I've been calling it the Monster City of the World, but if you look carefully on its birth certificate, there it is in ink: 'New York, the City of the Human Condition'. Its father is the Spirit of Man and its mother is America.

I realized something about New York once. It was that any description you might choose to put on it would be true – except for mountain ranges, miniature golf courses and shepherds. As a cab driver I've encountered people from every conceivable walk of life, but I must admit I've never met a shepherd. Why there are no miniature golf courses is a great mystery to me but, go figure, there's not a single one. And as for mountain ranges, the closest thing we've got is the mountain range of garbage that has accumulated on Staten Island – something you never want to be downwind of – but that doesn't count.

So you see what I'm getting at here. New York is a terrible place, New York is a wondrous place. It's filled with awfully rude people and it's filled with the nicest people you've ever met. Its joy will infect you, its misery will haunt you; there are saints, sinners and a church or a bar on nearly every block; it's where you go to soar, it's where you go to nose-dive from a bridge. Every variation of the human condition is not only represented, but well represented, here. New York is the human race. New York is the world.

55th between 8th and 9th

One summer evening in 1995 I picked up an older woman accompanied by a younger man who were coming from a theater in Union Square and heading to her apartment building on 55th Street between 8th and 9th Avenues. Both were nice people, quite conversational, and in talking with them I learned that the lady's name was Mary and that she was *ninety-nine and a half* years old (her proud words). I was thrilled because one of my very favorite kinds of fares is an elderly person who is still able to get around and enjoy living. But ninety-nine and a half! This was amazing! My own mother was seventy-seven at the time, and ailing, so I asked Mary, old enough to be my mother's mother, for advice.

'Be patient,' she said, after listening to my description of the difficulties I was encountering.

It turned out to be the most helpful guidance I could have wished for at that time and the memory of that ride has been a continual source of inspiration to me.

57th and 9th

It was around eleven o'clock on a November night in 1991 when I saw her coming toward me while I was stopped at a red light at 57th Street and 9th Avenue. She was one of the many beggars – homeless – mentally ill – derelicts – hustlers – that are always in the background in the scenery of New York City. It was hard to tell her age since the effects of substance abuse and the 'outdoor life' do much to add years to the appearance of a person, but I would have to say she was closer to seventy than fifty. She came right up to my window and tried the no-spin approach.

'Hey, mister cab driver,' she said, 'how about some change? I need a drink!'

I appreciated her honesty, but my personal policy of never giving money to panhandlers prevents me from making contributions, even if they're not trying to hide what it's all about. But I did feel some sympathy for her, so instead of a blunt 'sorry, no' without eye contact, I looked right at her with what I hoped would be perceived as an expression of empathy on my face.

'Sorry,' I said, trying not to sound too sanctimonious, 'but you're only killing yourself.'

She stood there for a moment to consider my comment. The expression on her face changed for just an instant and I thought maybe she'd had a memory of a time when things had been much better for her. But then the apathy came back and she started to turn to leave. Before she walked off, though, she said something to me.

'I'm already dead,' she said.

And then she disappeared into the night.

23rd between 6th and 7th

A middle-aged woman carrying a briefcase hailed me in Midtown at 3 a.m. on a frigid night in February, 2009. She wanted to make two stops – the first on 23rd Street between 6th and 7th Avenues and the second on Nassau Street in the Financial District. The briefcase told me she was going home from work and I began to automatically put her in that category in my mind, but there was something about her that didn't fit. It was her age. Briefcase equals someone who works in an office. But office workers going home at 3 a.m. are always twenty-somethings paying their dues at the bottom of the corporate ladder. She was too old for that, so it aroused my curiosity.

'So, are you a lawyer or a banker?' I asked. It had to be one or the other.

'A lawyer,' she said with a smile. 'How did you know?'

'You don't look like a bartender,' I replied.

My quip brought a smile to her face that remained there, inviting further conversation.

'Working late, huh?'

'Yes, it's been a long night.'

'Corporate stuff?'

'No, it's pro bono stuff tonight.'

She went on to tell me that she was a 'red tape navigator', helping homeless people find housing by preparing legal papers for the appropriate city and state agencies. I have a problem with the term 'homeless', so I asked her what kind of 'homeless' did she mean? Substance abusers? Mentally ill? She told me the people she was dealing with were those who'd lost their homes to foreclosures after the economic collapse in 2008 and had run out of safety nets. Unemployed, out of money, out of credit, out of friends or relatives who could take them in, they literally had no place to live.

I was startled by this. The only so-called 'homeless' people I ever encountered, and they were legion, were the junkies, hustlers and crazies who approached my cab seeking money. The truth is, it had never occurred to me that there could be people who were really just 'homeless'. This was a revelation.

Our first destination on 23rd Street turned out to be a church. Telling me she'd be less than a minute, she left the cab and knocked on a door, which immediately opened. As she spoke with the door-opener, I could see a hallway behind them in which people were sitting on chairs and appeared to be sleeping. After handing an envelope to this person, she returned to the cab and we headed downtown toward Nassau Street, where she lived.

I asked about the people in the hallway and was told that the church didn't have legal status as a shelter and therefore wasn't allowed to provide beds. So in lieu of that, people were permitted to sit on chairs and try to sleep. At least they were indoors. Again I was startled. I had become numb to seeing people sleeping on the streets of New York City, but the sight of people trying to sleep on chairs in the hallway of a church had a different effect on me. These weren't people who had given up on living, these were people who were trying to survive. If circumstances deteriorated sufficiently, it was not impossible to imagine that I could be sitting there, too.

As we continued the ride, our conversation free-flowing and effortless, my affinity and respect for my passenger increased. Here was a professional attorney who had stayed up half the night doing something effective for another person, probably someone she didn't even know, for no pay. Her kindness carried over in the way that she spoke to me, expressing gratitude that I would drive her home – something that was merely my job – and in the overly generous tip she bestowed upon me. I accepted the gratuity with a bit of guilt, thinking it might be more appropriate if I was tipping *her*, rather than the other way around.

There are certain people in this world whose basic goodness travels, osmosis-like, into those with whom they come into contact. After she had left my cab and I had waited on the street to make sure she made it into her building safely, some of that goodness seemed to have remained behind.

She had made me a better person.

29th *between* 7th *and* 8th

I had dropped off a passenger at Penn Station on a Sunday morning in June, 1983 and, finding no one there looking for my services, I decided to cruise down 7th Avenue to search for my next customer. I went only a couple of blocks before I was startled by a scary, shrill sound coming from my left. Scanning the area for its source, I saw that it was coming from a woman who was standing on the sidewalk screaming. Looking around for what could be causing such a commotion, I saw a man running as fast as he could across 7th Avenue, heading for 29th Street.

Reacting instinctively, as they say people do in these situations, I swerved the cab violently to the right and pursued this guy as he sprinted down 29th Street. As I began to catch up to him, I saw what had happened and what was about to happen. The man, really a kid because he couldn't have been more than twenty, was holding a woman's pocketbook under his arm. Obviously he had snatched it and now was making his big getaway. Waiting for him in the middle of the street was a parked car with a driver in it. So this was their modus operandi: the first guy grabs the pocketbook and the second guy drives them away.

As I caught up to the galloping thief in my cab, I found myself in a very peculiar situation. What should I do? Run him down?

No, of course I wouldn't do that, but I felt I had to do *something*. An idea presented itself – I could block the getaway car with my cab. It seemed like the right thing to do, so I pulled ahead and positioned the cab in such a way as to prevent the other car from going anywhere. Brilliant.

Uh, maybe not.

As the thief jumped into the getaway car and the driver saw that I was blocking him, he started honking his horn and yelling at me to get the hell out of his way. The thought occurred to me – and possibly it was because of this thought I lived to tell the tale – that a couple of guys who were crazy and stupid enough to be doing what they were doing might also be carrying a gun and be crazy and stupid enough to use it.

So I pulled out of the way, noting down the plate number and make of the car as they zoomed past me. They sped down 29th Street, made a right on 8th Avenue, and began zig-zagging through traffic. I gave chase from a safe distance for a few blocks, hoping to find a cop, which, of course, I did not. Finally I pulled over and called it in to 911 (no cell phones in those days).

Returning to the scene of the crime on 7th Avenue, I found the woman still there, apparently unharmed but in a state of shock, being comforted by a small group of strangers. I gave the information I had to one of the people attending to her and, being that I had a living to make, I went back to work.

The incident left me disgusted for a while at the quality of life, or lack of it, in the city, but it also left me with an insight. There were three or four seconds back there on 29th Street when I was right up next to the escaping mugger, three or four seconds in which I could observe him and get a feeling for what his reality was all about. And what I observed was this: that when this guy was in the act of committing his crime, he was as alive as he could be. The expression on his face was not one of apprehension or of rage at his personal demons. To the contrary, it was a huge grin, communicating that this – *this!* – was *fun.*

In his own way, he was in a state of perverted ecstasy. In the City of the Human Condition, that was the condition this particular person was in.

91st and Madison

They were a cheerful, elderly couple who were, if not octo-, then certainly septuagenarians. The gentleman was kind of like a teenager in an old man's body, full of mischief and fun, and his wife gave me the impression that she'd been his lifelong sidekick, laughing at his jokes and sometimes making him the object of her own, in a good-natured way.

Well, as you know, I love these rides with the elderly-active, and these two were a complete delight. They had just come from dinner at their son's place and were now on their way back to their own apartment. Sometimes parents are quite critical of or disappointed with the way their own offspring have turned out, but not these two.

'He's a good kid,' the gentleman said.

'How old is he?' I asked.

'Fifty-three.'

Sons and daughters are forever children in the eyes of their parents. We continued our chit-chat and general bonhomie until we arrived at their building at 91st Street and Madison Avenue. The elderly must be very careful, when exiting taxicabs, not to lose their footing as they step out onto the street, lest they slip and break a fragile bone. The gentleman walked with a cane, so

I was pleased when I saw that he'd made it to the sidewalk unscathed. As they waved goodbye, a nice gesture, the old man suddenly turned and called out to me.

'Hey, you want to see something?' he shouted. 'Take a look at this!'

And with that he pulled his cane apart, revealing an eight-inch dagger! With great delight, he proceeded to make stabbing motions with it into the air, sent an imaginary villain to his grave, and looked at me with a facial expression that seemed to say, "Yo, punk, you want a piece of me?" After a few more flails, he returned the weapon to its sheath and looked over at his wife for approval. She gave him one of those loving admonishments that mothers sometimes give to their misbehaving children, and then they both walked merrily down 91st Street and disappeared from sight.

Oh my God.

I'd just met the most dangerous man in New York City!

44th and 2nd

In the evening of September 27, 1982, I picked up a young corporate guy at 55th Street and 2nd Avenue who was going straight down 2nd to 17th. After telling me his destination, he pulled a newspaper out of his briefcase and buried his nose behind it, one way of signaling to the driver that he wasn't particularly interested in having a conversation. No problem, I don't expect every passenger to be conversational, so off we drove in silence.

The traffic on 2nd Avenue is usually free-flowing once you get below the 59th Street Bridge, but you never know for sure if that will be the case until you're actually there. Delays in the forms of double-parked trucks, gridlock on cross-town streets and backup from the Midtown Tunnel entrance down on 36th Street can pop up without warning. So I was annoyed but not surprised when the traffic suddenly ground to a halt at around 48th Street.

People usually ignore these delays until they've been sitting still for about a minute and notice that the pedestrians on the sidewalk are moving faster than they are. So when that minute had passed my passenger, right on cue, suddenly looked up and asked me what was going on. I wasn't sure, as this delay didn't yet fit into any category of known possibilities, and I was explaining this to him when we suddenly started moving again. There being no need for further elaboration, he returned to his newspaper and I returned to my navigation.

Our forward motion, however, was short-lived as we once again came to a stop at 46th Street. This time it took only half a minute for the guy's head to reappear and, as he asked again what I thought the problem was, I could already see from flashing lights in the distance that the source of the jam-up was some kind of police activity about two more blocks down the avenue. It happened to be 'UN Week' in the city, an annual event in which presidents and prime ministers from all over the world arrive at the United Nations building at 44th and 1st Avenue to address the General Assembly and hobnob with each other. It's always a time of sporadic traffic jams, so I told my passenger we were probably waiting for the president of Tierra del Fuego or somewhere to pass by. He seemed to understand.

We moved forward toward the source of the delay inch by inch, it seemed, and when we finally arrived at 44th Street I realized we weren't being delayed by a president, a prime minister or even a banana republic generalissimo.

We were being delayed by a riot!

Suddenly, like a new dream that is suddenly turned on in the middle of an existing one, we found ourselves quite literally in the middle of a scary brawl that was just on the verge of escalating into big time violence. On our right, behind a police barricade, were about a hundred demonstrators. One of them, a young man, for some reason had come out into the middle of 2nd Avenue and was resisting two cops who had wrestled him to the ground and were trying to put handcuffs on him. The demonstrators behind the barricade began chanting, 'Let him go! Let him go!' and then one of them ran through the police line to try to prevent the cops from making the arrest. More cops came running to assist the other cops. The crowd's chant increased in volume and was sounding like a group scream:

'Let him go!'

'Let him go!'

'Let him go!'

Some of the demonstrators, I could see, were trying to decide if they should break out and join in the fight themselves. A moment of truth was at hand.

While all this was happening, my cab sat at a dead standstill in the middle of the avenue. A cop stood right in front of me with his hand raised up in the 'stop' position. To his right, another cop was moving his arm back and forth as if to say, 'go', contradicting the other cop. A mounted horseman came galloping forward, billy club in hand, and I was close enough to him to observe the scariest thing yet – there was panic in his eyes. I knew instinctively that there could be gunfire at any moment.

I turned around to see how my passenger was doing and found him lying flat down on the floorboard in order to increase his chances of survival should the bullets indeed start flying. I considered doing the same, but thought better of it, which was a good thing because the cop who had been ordering me to stop had stepped out of the way and was now ordering me to go – which I did!

Bolting forward into what was now a 2nd Avenue devoid of any traffic, I was relieved to see that within three blocks of the incident, quite oddly, life was going on as normal. People were walking calmly on the sidewalk. A woman pushed a baby stroller across 41st Street.

'Wow, that was something,' I said to my passenger.

'Yeah, that was crazy,' he replied from behind his newspaper.

We arrived at his destination without further conversation. He paid me the fare, gave me an average tip, and, with his New York nonchalance intact, just went on his way as if nothing unusual had happened. I never found out what the furor had been all about – there was nothing about it in the papers or on TV.

It was just one of those mood swings the city is so capable of.

104th and Broadway

The night of November 4, 2008, was a night to remember no matter where you were in America. I was driving a cab in New York City.

Now, New York State, politically speaking, is thoroughly a 'blue state'. There was never any doubt which candidate was the favorite here and the national election was expected to go to the Democrats, but surveys are not results, of course, and you never know for sure who the winner will be until the votes are counted. It creates a certain amount of tension, but if the moods of my passengers had been a gauge of anticipation, you would have thought it was just another night. No one seemed too excited.

Until about half past eleven. I had just dropped off a passenger at 112th Street on the Upper West Side and was heading down Broadway in search of the next one. I got as far as 104th when I encountered a traffic jam caused by something I had never seen before in New York City – a spontaneous demonstration of joy at the announcement of the results of an election. A couple of hundred people had filled the intersection and were shouting in one voice:

'Yes we can!'

'Yes we can!'

'Yes we can!'

Barack Obama had been elected president of the United States.

To JFK

You certainly don't expect to get airport business at two o'clock in the morning. The last flights come in close to midnight and the first flights don't leave until around 6 a.m., leaving a gap in the middle of the night where there's nothing much going on out there. So my curiosity was immediately aroused when a young guy, college-aged, hailed me from in front of a Columbia University dorm at that early-morning hour in October, 1986, and told me he was going to Kennedy.

I was delighted. The streets had barely had a pulse for over an hour and the long ride to JFK was like winning twenty-five bucks on a scratch-off lottery ticket, or maybe like as if Fate had just pulled you aside, slipped some dough in your pocket, and whispered in your ear, 'You doin' awright, here, take dis, buy youself a new hat or somethin'.'

JFK at two in the morning – *yes!*

We put his luggage in the trunk and settled in for the thirty-five minute trip. First we had to get a little agreement on the route.

'I'm going to take the Triboro, okay?' I said. 'There's a toll on that bridge that you'll have to pay, but it's definitely the fastest way to go from here.' Taxi drivers are supposed to inform passengers about tolls before the ride begins.

'Okay,' he said.

That piece of business settled, we drove a block to Amsterdam Avenue and went up to 125th, the major cross-town street that leads into the Triboro. My joy at getting this unexpected fare overcame any inhibition I may have had about prying into why somebody would be going to Kennedy at this hour, so I dove right in.

'Where are you heading off to?' I asked.

'Louisville,' he replied softly.

'What airline?'

'It's a charter flight.'

'A charter flight to Louisville at 2 a.m. – wow, that's so unusual! What are you, a rock star or something?'

Looking at him in the mirror, his face seemed to crumble. 'My mother died,' he said, almost in a whisper. And then he burst into tears.

I was stunned, of course, and offered him the obligatory 'I'm sorry'. But I could find no other words of solace for the young man, no words that would seem appropriate at a time like this. We made the ride to JFK in silence, the solemnity of the journey interrupted only by the occasional sound of his weeping.

I wished, instead of leaving him in a dark and deserted airport, I could have taken him to a prearranged location, maybe a Chinese restaurant somewhere, where he'd find it had all been one of Fate's stupid little jokes. His mother was actually alive and well, saving a seat for him at the table, and wondering what had taken him so long to get there.

Why do people have to die?

From JFK

I had been waiting in the taxi lot at American Airlines for half an hour or so on a pleasant evening in June, 1990, when suddenly the line started moving – two flights had come in simultaneously and the newly arriving passengers were jumping out of the terminal like popcorn popping. Within five minutes one of them was sitting in the back seat of my cab and we were on our way, fortunately, to Manhattan. (When you pick up a fare at the airport, you're always a little worried that the ride will be a shortie to Brooklyn or Queens. Manhattan is the place you want to go.)

My passenger was a barely twenty-something kid, an Agoger, eyes all aglow at coming to the Big Apple for the very first time. New York was the place he'd been dreaming of coming to forever, he said, and finally his dream was coming true. He was from the Midwest somewhere and had studied documentary filmmaking at a bunch of different schools, and now at last it was time to take the Big Plunge. I could feel the excitement of his anticipation although we were still ten miles away from the part of New York that even New Yorkers call 'the city'… *Manhattan.*

You know, I have been saying that one of my favorite kinds of fares is the one with elderly people who are still enjoying living. Let me confide in you now that my *very* favorite type of ride - the one at the top of the list – is this one, the trip into Manhattan with the wide-eyed virgin, so to speak. I become the impromptu tour guide, an embedded guru, offering advice and insider skinny, but secretly longing to experience vicariously the thrill I hope they are about to have when they see *it* for the very first time.

After twenty minutes of stop and go on the Long Island Expressway we arrived at the last exit you can take before entering the Midtown Tunnel – I did *not* want to take that route into the city – and I got off there. We drove a few more blocks and soon arrived at the exact spot where I wanted to be for this particular ride – the entrance to the Upper Level of the 59th Street Bridge on Thomson Street. I made a right onto the long ramp that rises, before it feeds onto the bridge, above houses, factories and the Number Seven subway line. There are five bridges that span the East River, but the one with not only the best view, but the best *feel*, is the Upper Level of the 59er, and that's why I chose to take him this way. I wanted him to feel it.

Now here's the thing about the Upper Level – first, the broad skyline, that endless vista of skyscrapers – is one of the great sights of the world. You can see many of New York's iconic structures quite clearly, and that in itself is spectacular, but the main thing, due to its location and its clear sightlines, is the sense you have of the city getting larger and larger and LARGER as you approach it. New York, that far away dream, is becoming a reality. Look – *look!* – there it is! It's really there! And then, as the roadway of the bridge begins to descend toward ground level, the immensity of the place starts to sink in, the buildings gradually seem to surround you – *look, you can see people inside them!* – and one has the sense of being literally devoured by Gotham. Finally touching down on East 62nd Street, the energy level of New York City immediately hits you in the face. People are crowding the street, walking quickly as if they're late for something, the traffic is bumper to bumper, and, hey, look at that – there really *are* yellow taxicabs all over the place!

I studied my passenger in the mirror. He was gazing eagerly out his window, trying to take it all in, mesmerized and enchanted, as I hoped he would be.

'So what do you think?' I asked.

'Wow!' was all he could say.

I was delighted, but I was not done. We headed across town on 63rd Street, made a left on 5th Avenue, and started coasting down the avenue that divides Manhattan into east and west.

'Look,' I said, 'there's Central Park.'

'Wow!'

'There's Tiffany's.'

'Wow!'

'There's St Patrick's Cathedral.'

'Wow!'

'There's Rockefeller Center.'

'Wow!'

When we got to the south side of 34th Street, I suddenly pulled over to the curb and stopped.

'Get out,' I commanded.

He was confused. 'Get out?'

'Yes, get out and look up.'

He did as he was told and found himself looking straight up at the tallest building he had ever seen. You just can't appreciate the size and the magnificence of the Empire State Building unless you're standing right under it.

'Oh my God!' he exclaimed as he climbed back into the cab. He smiled like a little kid at his own birthday party who was about to start opening a whole roomful of presents.

Oh, yes. He had arrived.

It had begun.

89th and WEA

I was finishing up my shift at around 5 a.m. on a Saturday night in June, 1993, the time when the first rays of sunlight begin breaking through on the horizon. If you drive a cab at this hour, you will see two types of people on the street – those whose night is ending and those whose day is beginning.

As I came to a stop at a red light at 89th Street and West End Avenue, two such people suddenly appeared in the middle of the intersection. Correction – two such people *and a horse,* a magnificent, thoroughbred-looking animal mounted by a mustachioed, Teddy Roosevelt kind of man who wore a wide-brimmed hat pulled up on one side. He was the picture of the rugged outdoorsman and what in the world he and his horse were doing on the Upper West Side of Manhattan at this (or any other) hour was utterly weird and a complete mystery to me. But there he was.

Not to be outdone in the realm of the bizarre, however, was a lone pedestrian who appeared from out of nowhere and took his place in the middle of the avenue. Apparently a drunk on his way home from a long night of overdoing it, he at first just stood there, his marinated brain attempting to comprehend what was standing in front of him. Then, after a few moments of computation, he realized what he must do: he must ridicule the horse. Walking right up to the animal and sticking his face within biting distance, he bared his teeth, bobbed his head up and down, and began a long and repetitive neigh that was clearly intended not to praise, but to demean the noble beast. To add to the insult, he then went into a sarcastic, circular strut, continuing the obnoxious neighing and flapping his arms around like a chicken.

Well, the horseman was not going to let it pass. He stared down at the fool with a look of contempt that seemed to say 'you can malign me, but you cannot – you *cannot,* sir – malign my horse!', and he began to dismount. The joker antagonist, not big on macho pride, immediately turned and ran to the sidewalk with a look of mock, wide-eyed terror on his face and then stood there waiting to see what the horseman, now off the charger and standing in the middle of West End Avenue with the reins in his hand, would do. Apparently satisfied that he had caused the guy to make a cowardly retreat, he remounted and began to trot away.

But it wasn't over. The joker, realizing the horseman wasn't really able do anything to him because he couldn't release his grip on the reins, jogged back onto West End Avenue and resumed his neighing. The horseman swung his horse around, confronting him. The joker backed off, but just a few feet this time, and continued to taunt the horseman with a few more neighs. And then…

… the light turned green.

Needing to get back to my garage quickly for fear that I would have to pay the day shift driver for lost time, I circled around the combatants and continued downtown on West End Avenue. Cruising along, I wondered if maybe a couple of those funny mushrooms had been slipped into my salad and the whole thing had been an hallucination.

But no, there had been no mushrooms.

It had just been a New York minute.

72nd between CPW and Columbus

On a Friday evening in July, 1979, three young fellows dressed in the colorful costumes of medieval Europe jumped in on 72nd Street between Central Park West and Columbus Avenue. They were Spanish troubadours carrying with them the tools of their trade – a guitar, a mandolin, and what I assumed was a lute – who were coming from the El Faro 72 restaurant right there on 72nd where, they said, they had just entertained the diners for the last hour. And now it was on to another restaurant in Little Italy.

I pulled out from the curb and we headed downtown.

They told me they were students at a university in Madrid and that keeping the traditional music of Spain alive was a common activity among the young people back home. The fact that they were doing it in New York was due to two things: they needed summer jobs and they were good.

'Oh, you're good, huh?' I said, pretending to be skeptical. 'Okay, let's hear it.'

They needed no further encouragement. For the remainder of the ride I was an audience of one in my own little yellow concert hall. Gliding melodiously down Broadway, it must have created quite a scene to anyone who happened to notice us go by – a cab driver being serenaded by three guys from the Middle Ages.

It wasn't long after that ride that I stopped looking through the help-wanted pages. New York City Taxi Driver was to be my profession.

43rd and Lex

I was sitting in my cab on East 43rd Street, facing Lexington Avenue, on a September evening in 1982, waiting for the light to turn green. I didn't have a passenger in the taxi, but I figured I would soon be getting one as it was the rush hour and I was within spitting distance of Grand Central Station, a great place to find a fare. I relaxed behind the wheel and was rather blankly observing the stream of people and vehicles hurrying on by.

Suddenly appearing before me on Lex was an astonishing sight: a young man dressed in a business suit was riding a bicycle, and he was moving along quite rapidly. He appeared to be a commuter on his way home from work, but, aside from the fact that he was on a bicycle, there was something else that set him apart from the other passersby on the avenue – it was a dog, a wirehaired terrier, who was *standing* with his rear legs on an attaché case that had been fastened to the bike just behind the seat, while his front legs were resting on the young man's back, almost as if he were steering him. Unattached by leash or harness, the dog was completely on his own, a consummate acrobat, and with his face turned toward me as they went zipping by, I could see that he was literally grinning from ear to doggy ear, sending out a picture of complete exhilaration.

They appeared and disappeared in five seconds, to be replaced once again by the mundane. Yet this image – so instant, so unexpected, so joyful – has remained fresh in my mind for all these years. It wound up becoming my own personal metaphor for this thing that is known as New York City. And it can be your metaphor, too, if you'd like. I wanted to pass that along to you now that we've reached the end of our ride.

On the left or the right over here?

There you go.

Thanks for paying in cash. I'm not a big fan of these credit card machines.

Careful as you get out – better use the curb side, it's the law. Be a pity to lose you now! Be a pity to lose my door, too.

See ya.

Hey, wait. You know, there's one other thing I'd like to share with you before you're back on foot, a little taxi driver homily, if I may – my tip to you! It's a point of view thing.

You know, I know I've been digressing here about New York, and I mentioned something a little bit back there about the city's gravitational pull and something about how, internalizing its challenges, one could 'master it'. I want to let you know what I meant by that.

Now, it's not like you don't know this already. I just think it's one of those things that it's good to be reminded of every once in a while. Okay, it's like this. Your reality is *your* reality – you own it. You don't have to go into agreement with somebody else's reality. That's the challenge. What's unique about New York is that you

can do this and not feel like you're an outsider. I've often said that there are no foreigners in this city. No one feels like they don't belong here. And it's true.

The way I see it, at least on my better days, is that New York is basically a gigantic playground and the objects, structure, and even the people are all there for you to decide how they fit into your own personal scheme of things. Looking at it that way, a street, for example, might not be just a street but a perfectly suitable place for 'the dance'. If you will permit me to wax poetic here, you might say Broadway is for the boogaloo, Madison is for the mambo, and First is for the fandango. It's up to you. If you want them to be that, then they *are* that.

Taking this a step further, parks are for poetry – how about William Butler Yeats at the break of dawn? Oh, all right then, at the break of noon. Bridges are for brunching on and watching tugboats tugging from. Libraries are for lounging in and cops are for complimenting on the way they wear their hats. (Or for completely avoiding if you're carrying any contraband, of course.)

Let's see… buses are for bouncing on your butt in the back seat in. Elevators are for doing animal imitations in with a friend until someone else enters the car, in which case you would do them silently with facial expressions, unless the person entering the car is also doing animal imitations, in which case you could all keep doing them out loud.

Subways, you might have heard, are for sleeping. But today you can get a summons if you fall asleep in a subway, so we'd better change that. How about subways are for finger frolicking in with or without finger puppets while listening to Beethoven's Fifth on your iPod? Sounds good. Statues are for saluting at, very seriously, you know, and museums are for marching through in certain secret waltzes past the dinosaurs, the Van Goghs and the early Indian artifacts.

I think we've covered a lot of ground here. What else is there? Is there something commonly associated with New York City that I've failed to mention? Perhaps something in yellow?

Ah, yes – cabs!

Cabs – what do you suppose they could be for? Hey, I know the answer to that one.

Cabs are for kissing.

Acknowledgments

Thank you to the readers of my blog for your attention and kind words.

Thank you to my fellow taxi driver bloggers around the world for your attention and kind words, too. It's a club of which I'm proud to be a member.

Thank you to friends and family for your advice and support, particularly Nikki Armstrong, Ann Devert, Marcy Gordon and my daughter Susanna Salomon.

Thank you to Scott Pack, my editor and publisher at The Friday Project, for your patience, guidance, wit and brilliance. Scott's blog, Me And My Big Mouth (http://meandmybigmouth.typepad.com), is the place to go for expert insight about what's going on in the world of books.

Thank you most of all to friend and fellow blogger Jodie Schofield, a Liverpool lass, without whose help this book might never have come to pass. Visit the Jodester's blog, Don't Panic, at http://jodesters.blogspot.com.

And thank you to you, dear reader, for coming along for the ride. You have an open invitation to join me again at my own blog, Cabs Are For Kissing, at http://cabsareforkissing.blogspot.com. Until then…

May your best days be yet unseen,
And may all your lights be green.